Praise for
CHILD'S PLAY

"*Child's Play* is an inspirational, practical book that every parent should read. Of course, we should expect nothing less from Silken Laumann."

—Russ Kisby, former president
of ParticipACTION

"Laumann's book is a practical approach about encouraging activity and unstructured play in almost any community. Her flashbacks to her childhood days of free play and the value of these experiences, even to a woman who would later become a competitive athlete, not only make sense but make one take a second look."

—Urbanmoms.ca

"Our Olympians are powerful role models for youth, and in *Child's Play* Silken Laumann has eloquently reminded all of us of the power of sport and play to transform the lives of our children. I share Silken's vision and believe that the human legacy of healthy, active and inspired kids is the best legacy we can have."

—John Furlong, Chief Executive Officer, Vancouver
Organizing Committee for the 2010 Olympic
and Paralympic Winter Games

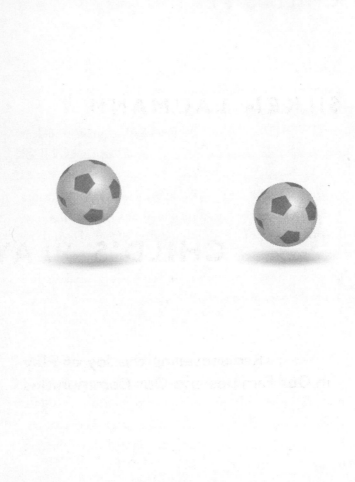

SILKEN LAUMANN

May 07

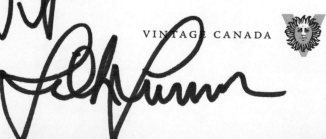

CHILD'S PLAY

Jennifer ,

Rediscovering the Joy of Play
in Our Families and Our Communities

*Let's keep our kids
joyful and active.*

VINTAGE CANADA

VINTAGE CANADA EDITION, 2007

Copyright © 2006 Silken & Co. Productions Ltd.

Published in Canada by Vintage Canada, a division of Random House of Canada Limited, Toronto, in 2007. Originally published in hardcover in Canada by Random House Canada, a division of Random House of Canada Limited, Toronto, in 2006. Distributed by Random House of Canada Limited, Toronto.

Vintage Canada and colophon are registered trademarks of Random House of Canada Limited.

www.randomhouse.ca

LIBRARY AND ARCHIVES CANADA CATALOGUING IN PUBLICATION

Laumann, Silken, 1964–

    Child's play : rediscovering the joy of play in our families
and our communities / Silken Laumann.

Includes bibliographical references and index.

ISBN 978-0-679-31407-3

    1. Child development. 2. Child rearing. 3. Games. 4. Play. 5. Physical education for children. 6. Sports for children. I. Title.

HQ782.L36 2007   649'.5   C2006-904704-9

Cover and text design: CS Richardson

Printed and bound in Canada

10 9 8 7 6 5 4 3 2 1

For my children:
   Sweet William, You see the truth in the world
   and help us all see more clearly.

   Kate,
   You are like a brilliant firework, spreading a million bits
   of light into every corner of your world.

   I love you both, beyond words

CONTENTS

Be the change you want to see in the world.

MAHATMA GANDHI

THE DREAM

Not long ago, on a damp, fall evening, my children, Kate and William, and I were taking our thirteen-year-old golden retriever, Banner, on a quick lap around the block before dinner. As I neared the dead-end road by my neighbourhood park, I heard the distinctive *thwack* of a hockey stick on asphalt. *Slam* went the stick, *whack* went the ball—the sound was rhythmic and constant as my young neighbour Mark slapped his bright orange hockey puck into the net over and over again. A car came up behind us, and Mark glided over to pick up the net so the car could pass. He moved the net effortlessly back again and resumed his play, oblivious to my watching eyes.

Hearing that sound of stick on pavement transported me back to the noisy streets of my childhood. On the roads I grew up on, there was always a group of kids playing street shinny and screaming, "Pass, pass, pass!"

Unlike many other Canadians I've met, hockey wasn't my passion—I loved capture-the-flag. In my neighbourhood we played this game almost obsessively. The objective, as the name implies, was to capture the other team's marker "flag." But if you were caught on the other team's territory, you were "frozen" and had to wait to be rescued by one of your teammates. I would call, "I'm frozen, I'm frozen!" at the top of my lungs, hand stretched out, craning and leaning until someone on my team managed to sprint across enemy lines to release me. We would play non-stop until a parent finally shouted, "Dinner!"

Kids used to live outside. Adventure was a central part of most days, found in the form of a scavenger hunt down a path near home, a trip to the neighbourhood Mac's Milk, a meeting of friends on the first snowy day to sneak our toboggans onto the exhilaratingly steep slopes of the Mississauga golf course.

—

I must have been staring at Mark for a while, lost in thought, because he eventually looked up at me curiously. I smiled and move on. The streets my children and I walk resemble the ones I grew up on—snug houses, big old trees and tons of space for adventures—but there is one critical difference: the streets today are silent. Mark was the only kid I saw that evening. The playground we dodged through was empty, and so were the schoolyard and all the driveways we passed. And it was *so* quiet; there was a notable absence of boisterous shouting and gleeful laughter.

I miss these children who make too much noise, whose fluorescent orange hockey balls get too close to my car window. I miss their energy, their smiles, and I miss the community these kids help create. I remember the neighbourhoods of my childhood and can't help but compare them to my neighbourhood now. Those streets and parks and play spaces were ours.

Children have disappeared from our streets, seemingly overnight. Some are inside their homes, where television, the computer and video games entertain them for hours on end. Others stay in after-school care until their busy parents return from work, or are shuttled to prearranged lessons. In a busy world, where parents are under an almost unbearable pressure to balance work, family and their own health, quality family time is often snatched in the minivan on the way to hockey practice, or in the few moments before bedtime.

Even a decade ago, kids still played in the parks and streets of their community after school. They met with friends and learned to skip in the driveways; their mom or dad might have come outside for a quick game of soccer or basketball. While the kids played, parents grabbed a piece of sanity and that necessary half-hour to prepare dinner. My mom made dinner in peace while the three of us kids played outside.

> Play is the lifeblood of childhood—it brings children joy, it nurtures and excites their creativity, it builds social skills and it strengthens their bodies.

People say the world has changed: our streets aren't safe, kids can't go outside alone and parents don't have the time to watch their kids play in a neighbourhood park. I try to accept this logic and yet I can't help but believe that the way we are living today isn't really working. We are denying children the best and most vital part of childhood: play. Play is the lifeblood of childhood—it brings children joy, it nurtures and excites their creativity, it builds social skills and it strengthens their bodies. Play is the very best part of being a kid. I can't accept that something so good for their hearts and minds and bodies, something so good for us as parents, has been lost.

Children may have more toys and more treats and fancier bicycles, but they have lost much of the freedom that made our childhoods so joyful. A good friend of mine grew up in Rycroft, a tiny northern Alberta village. His single mom supported her four children by cutting hair in the daytime and slinging beer at night. There wasn't much time for cuddles, and yet Paul remembers his childhood as happy. Why? He had the love of a parent and the luxury of spending all his free time outdoors, riding his bicycle, finding friends and playing kick-the-can or intense games of road hockey.

I began to ask *why* things have changed and *how* things have changed, why we seem to be okay or at least resigned to this change and whether or not I was alone in my desire to reconnect with the past. I started to dream of my neighbourhood as a place where my kids could meet in the park, where they could roam the streets with their buddies on bikes or skateboards or scooters, where there would be a championship road-hockey game in my driveway.

I began to dream about *how* I could make this possible, not *if* it was possible. I decided that I couldn't be alone in this—my neighbourhood is full of parents my age, parents who would have grown up playing as I did, full-tilt until dinner. I knew that moving to a different neighbourhood was not the answer—the solution had to be about creating opportunities for kids to play right here on my streets. And I couldn't wait for someone else to come along and take the initiative for me; if I was unsatisfied with my neighbourhood, then I had to do something to change it.

If I wanted my kids to play in the park, why not invite some local kids to come and play with them one night a week?

The idea, when it came, was so simple: if I wanted my kids to play in the park, why not invite some local kids to come and play with them one night a week? Surely I could find a few other willing parents to help me supervise—perhaps we could even dig up some soccer balls, some sidewalk chalk, badminton rackets . . . even a pogo stick or two! It seemed pretty doable, and as I began talking to my neighbours about letting their children play once a week together, I found I was met with considerable enthusiasm. *That's a great idea.*

If nothing else, parenting has turned me into an acute observer. At the same time as I realized that my family's quality of life needed to change, I began to notice the general physical condition of the kids around me.

At the pool, I noticed how many kids were over-weight or obese; I noticed how many girls hid their heavy bodies under T-shirts; I noticed how many boys got teased for being chubby. I was troubled to see a nine-year-old totally winded after climbing the stairs to the waterslide. I saw parents of average weight holding the hands of children who were clearly overweight, and wondered how that could be. I compared the kids I was seeing now to the kids I grew up with and could not recall such a high proportion of out-of-shape and overweight kids. In my class, there was one child who was considered "fat." One. I consulted some prominent Canadian studies and was shocked to learn that today almost 40% of children are overweight or obese. This statistic corresponded with what I was seeing, but I still had trouble accepting a number that high.

With an issue as complex as systemic childhood obesity and overweight, it is not possible to locate one cause to heap all the blame on, despite our natural urge to find a scapegoat for every problem. Yet I did see a link between the unexpected stillness of living in a neighbourhood filled with kids and the current state of our children's bodies. I understood that link to be a place where I could focus my energy, where my dream of kids screaming through the neighbourhood could have a larger impact on the physical and mental health of our kids and maybe even change the way we live in our communities.

If anyone had said to me then that I was on the verge of beginning a "social movement," I would have laughed in polite disbelief. Social movements are the products of enormous energy and resources; they are political and revolutionary, not the result of a concerned mother who just wants to see more kids playing . . . right?

I have been extremely fortunate to have some positive role models in my life, people who have helped me believe that each one of us has something wonderful to give this world. My friend Rick Hansen has always shined in this way—his passion for spinal cord research and belief in a cure for spinal cord injury and degeneration eventually led to the Rick Hansen Institute, an association that has raised millions of dollars to improve the lives of people affected by spinal cord injuries and disease.

In April 2004, on a plane bound for New York, I happened to meet another person I now consider a role model—a man by the name of Ric Young. We were both on our way to a Right to Play conference and struck up a conversation. He asked me lots of questions about what I was doing, about my passion for kids, about my belief that so many of the problems with kids' health could be prevented by providing opportunities for them to play. Ric views the world through the lens of social change, and he helped me to see our conversation as part of a vision that a lot of us share, part of the unexpressed longing of many, many people: a longing for community and connection and kids all over our streets.

As we spoke, I reflected on a talk I had given for a series called Leadership for Kids' Sake in Waterloo, Ontario, about three years earlier. I remembered that I had chosen to focus my speech on play and community, and how I believe we can re-create the neighbourhoods that used to allow and even encourage kids to safely engage in unstructured play. I talked about the childhood I had known, shared some of my favourite memories of playing, elaborated on the benefits of having such an active childhood. I spoke to a crowd of thirteen hundred, and when it was over, about half of the audience came up to me to share their own memories of playing. That was all the encouragement I needed to know I was on to something. Even now, when I mention this book to others, they almost always lapse into a happy memory of playing hockey on a frozen pond in Saskatchewan, toes freezing, but soldiering on in order to get one more game in. They recall games of kick-the-can and laugh about the rules they used to make up and then change and then change again. I watch as people are taken back to that magical time when their neigh-bourhoods held all the adventure they could dream up and there was always someone to play with. What saddens me is when they finish off by saying, in a half-resigned, half-baffled voice, "Kids don't do that any-more—it's sad."

Sad, yes; acceptable, no. That conversation with Ric made me realize how passionate I am about the power of play and recognize my unswerving commit-ment to my belief that every child deserves to play. Every child must have that opportunity. Ric helped me to hear the anger and frustration in my voice when I talked about how unhealthy our kids are becoming, how parents allow their kids to watch endless hours of TV or spend the whole night play-ing computer games. My voice started to rise when I talked about what kids need to be physically, emo-tionally and spiritually healthy. Ric also got me to acknowledge the privileged position I am in as some-one who has the opportunity to influence people on this issue, and the responsibility I have to do just that: "You really care about this, Silken. I think you are going to do something about it."

I just couldn't accept that my kids would never be able to walk to school alone, or ride their bikes with their friends, or explore the park together. The independence and joy my children would gain from the freedom to explore their community is so precious I knew I simply had to do something to make it possible. I needed to recognize what was no longer working for me or my kids and find solutions that do work. I have a card on my desk that reads, "Be the change you want to see in the world." Gandhi's words seem appropriate and heroic when applied to ending world hunger and working for world peace. Could the change *I* want to see in the world begin with walking a group of kids to school, creating unstructured play in my park and connecting with neighbours to help supervise a playground?

It can be difficult to see past what is. We can become so overwhelmed by "now" that we forget that we are the ones who shape today and tomorrow. Only fifteen years ago, kids spent most of their time outdoors. Now many go *days* where the only outside time they get is between the car and the house, or the bus and the next scheduled activity. We don't see kids on the street, so it is hard to imagine that our streets could be filled with children again. Change starts by passionately believing that what exists is not good enough. I want to be part of a community where children play in the parks and driveways and schoolyards. I want our children to be vibrant and healthy, to have energy and imagination and a sense of community. I want to live in a country whose greatest strength is the relationship between its citizens, where we know each other and watch each other's kids, where we meet in the common spaces of our neighbourhoods to talk and share our joys and challenges.

This is my dream for all of us and especially for our kids. This dream is motivating me to make changes on behalf of my children, and this dream is sustaining me in the face of what is "now."

The incredible thing about "now" is that it's fleeting, it's dynamic, and that means it's ready for change. Right now, family time is being stolen by the sheer pace of our lives and the vortex created by the many screens in our homes: the television screen, the computer screen, the video screen. On a Friday night when I come home exhausted and unable to think straight, letting the kids watch a movie can help me gain the strength for round two: bath and bedtime. But our kids watch too much television. Most of us know it, but we need to take that knowledge and develop a plan—a plan that reflects what we want in our families and communities. We can use our imaginations to see a different way of being in a family, where the TV or computer does not dominate and shape how we spend our time together—a way of living where we don't rush through dinners because a program's coming on or a computer game needs to be taken to the next level.

It is so easy to slip into these nights in front of our television set, or to a constant stream of evenings spent rushing to our children's lessons and our own commitments. And it is even tough to imagine how it could be different.

But that evening walk around my own neighbourhood reminded me of what is possible.

I think about this simple act of exploring the neighbourhood with my children, of waving to people as they drive by, of watching the dog bound through a neighbour's yard, my children racing after her yelling, "No, Banner, no!" I feel close to my family and a part of this neighbourhood; I can hear the pulse of it; I have time to see all the things I don't notice while driving. My kids whined and complained before we left the house, but now they are running and jumping, fresh air clearing their heads and lungs. We walk for twenty minutes, and for the last ten my eight-year-old holds my hand. He tells me about the spelling test he had and the words he got wrong; he points to the moon and asks me when it will be full again; he remarks at how fast his little sister now runs. I wish we could stay still in this moment, his little hand pressed in mine, as we both take in the beautiful evening.

These evening walks are the stuff of memories, my children's and mine, and they are, without a doubt, the beautiful moments in the tough job of parenting. These are moments of my own childhood replaying before my eyes. My fondest memories of my parents are of the times we walked and talked together. The fresh air seemed to open me up and make me more receptive to questions about school and friends. When my dad and I visit now, we almost always go for a walk together, because that is how we do our best talking and connecting. By taking the time and energy to go outside with our children to explore a local park, by stopping for a minute together to observe a dragonfly, we are developing the memories of childhood that last a lifetime. I also believe these will become the memories of parenting that linger long after my kids leave home—they will be what I think about when I miss them; they will become stories I share with their kids.

Our kids are worth it ... Individually and collectively, we can create a family life and communities that will give our kids a better and more empowering childhood experience.

Our kids are worth it. They are worth the effort of challenging what is. Individually and collectively, we can create a family life and communities that will give our kids a better and more empowering childhood experience. We can create environments that better equip our children to be engaged and creative members of our society. I see it happening all around me, including in my assistant's three kids, who play basketball outside before breakfast, who run and dance and use their imaginations for hours of unstructured play every week. Laurie has given them that gift by making play a priority in their family.

There are tremendous pressures working against us: Xbox, Nintendo, non-stop children's programming on TV, and the ever-present computer bidding for our children's time and attention. And then there is the pressure of giving our kids a "headstart"—music lessons at age three, soccer practice at four, hockey leagues at five. There is a part of most parents that is afraid of missing some ill-defined window for our child's greatness. What if our child could have been a great musician if she had only started piano lessons earlier? It is this insecurity that pushed me to sign up both my kids up for piano before any of us were ready. I know what is competing for our children's time— most of us do—but it doesn't make what is happening to our children and to our communities accept-able. I will not allow our children's quality of life to continue to erode. I want kids to experience personal freedom, connection to community, and ample opportunity to run around and be kids. Most impor-tantly, I will not have precious family time taken away from me: it is not negotiable time, because that's when I get to be with them—when we play together, when we get to walk hand in hand.

I look at our schools and I know we can all do better in this area as well. Our schools can and should be places where teachers, administrators and parents are deeply committed to developing the whole child—mind, body and spirit. Our schools can be an extension of our families and the epicentre of the communities we want. How did we get to a place in our schools where we emphasize our children's minds and let their bodies fall by the wayside? We know that when a body is healthy the mind thinks more clearly, but we have allowed physical education and activity to be cut out of our school curriculums and budgets. We are focusing so intensely on academics that we have forgotten that our children need to move, that they actually learn through movement and that they experience greater joy and self-esteem and excitement for school when physical activity is part of their daily routine there.

Active children have lower rates of drug and alcohol abuse, and girls who continue to play sport have a far lower chance of teenage pregnancy.

—

When our children move, they learn to see their bodies as beautiful creations, deserving of respect and care. "Look at me skip!" shouts my eight-year-old neighbour Sage as we turn the rope singing, "Cinderella, Dressed in Yellow." "Did you see me get the ball?" asks my son at the weekend's soccer game. These children are taking pride in their skills and movements, and developing a vital connection to their bodies. I wish for these children to keep moving their bodies through to adulthood. I know that if they do, they will come to feel personal power in their bodies and to understand that their physicality is not separate from their intellect and spirit. This connection will help them make better decisions about their bodies. Active children have lower rates of drug and alcohol abuse, and girls who continue to play sport have a far lower chance of teenage pregnancy.

Our school system disrespects our children's bodies by ignoring their physical needs on a daily basis. This is a strong statement, but it is a reflection of what is happening in far too many of our schools. Children are not given daily physical education, and they are being taught PE by generalist teachers who often have little if any training in this area. Parents have not advocated for better quality and greater quantity of activity, and in a stretched curriculum, physical education has fallen to the low end of the priority list. My son said to me, "I like school, but we have to sit all the time. Why can't we have more play time?" I don't have an answer for him that makes sense; I know that greater amounts of play time would help him enjoy school more, would improve his concentration and would make him a more eager and alert student, so I can't justify a system that makes him sit still for most of the day. His school is, however, working hard to make changes that will give children far more opportunities to be physically active within the classroom and in the gym. It has a dedicated PE teacher, and the school principal and staff are commited to introducing more activity into the day. They have begun a fifteen-minute exercise and dance warm-up each morning before classes begin. It's inspiring to see what a little effort can do. But in order for these changes to occur in *all* our schools, we need to empower the teachers with ideas and workshops, and parents' support is critical. We must be the voices for our children's physical and mental health. We must ask for environments within our schools that give kids outdoor time, we must empower our teachers to teach physical education with training and confidence, and we must create food policies that offer only healthy choices.

I dream that one day our schools will be places

where the physical health of our children is a high priority. I dream of a community where our kids can play outside, walk to school and gather in a safe place to enjoy unstructured play and let their imaginations run wild. We want our children to have the same great childhood memories we did—admittedly, they won't be *exactly* the same memories; the park may be supervised by a neighbour or two, and there may be a lawn chair parked beside the game of road hockey or (even better) a parent playing the game with them. Our world has changed, but it can still have that beautiful element of children coming together to play—children of different ages and genders, without rules and referees, without structure and constrictions—playing for the sheer fun of it.

The power of dreaming has been very real in my life. Never was this power more evident than in 1992, after my accident in Germany ten weeks before the Olympic games. During practice, I was broadsided by a men's pair. Their boat crashed into mine, and my boat splintered, driving hundreds of pieces of razor-sharp wood into my right lower leg, shredding muscles, damaging nerves and bones and causing extensive skin damage. In the days following my accident, a doctor told me that I would not row at the Olympic level again. He was basing his prognosis on what he had seen in his practice and on the extent of my injuries. For a few days after my accident, I was overwhelmed by his statement and by the obvious severity of the injury. I was grappling with the enormity of what had just happened and trying to imagine how I would get better. I knew I had to have a dream—a dream of getting out of this hospital bed, a dream of walking and rowing again, a dream that could help me not succumb to the enormity of the obstacles I was facing.

The dream of going to the Olympics in ten weeks' time, of winning a medal—this dream defied my present reality: a bandaged leg, broken ankle and extensive skin grafts. Yet this dream is what gave me the energy and passion to move past seemingly insurmountable obstacles.

During the weeks of operations and physiotherapy, training and recovery, belief sustained my dream. At the deepest centre of my being, I truly believed that competing at the Olympics—heck, *winning a medal*—was possible. It wasn't rational, logical or realistic, but I believed it. How many times in our lives has belief anchored our dreams? We believe all the time in things we have no evidence for. We take courses because we want to be better parents, we read books and consult experts to become more capable in our work, we learn by doing, all the time believing that we are getting better, that we bring more to our lives each day. Can we measure how we are progressing? For most dreams, we can't step on the track and time ourselves over a mile and see quite clearly that we are one second faster than we were last year at this time. No, we invest ourselves in our dreams each day, but sometimes we have to wait years for proof of our progress.

As parents we need this kind of belief. We need to take action on behalf of our kids, in our families, in our schools and in our communities. The change may take a little while. What I have proof of already, though, is that lots of people are worrying about our kids: community champions, schools and governments are already taking action. Now we must add our efforts to those around us and create what Malcolm Gladwell calls a "tipping point"—a point where so many of us are helping get kids active, so many of us are making changes in our families and helping our schools be places where kids are active and healthy, that change comes faster and faster and becomes more far-reaching.

I know I can't change my community alone, but I am discovering I don't have to. When I asked if my neighbours would help supervise the local park, they took over the initiative so I could focus on getting more parks in my area started. My heroes are ordinary people. They are moms and dads and social workers and teachers whom I have met on this journey to help get kids active. They are people like Verlee Hagley, from the tiny town of Rouleau, Saskatchewan. Verlee opened the community high school in the evening and invited everyone to come in from the cold prairie winter to play floor hockey and dodge ball, or even learn how to cook a healthy meal. About half the town now comes into that school every Wednesday night. Or Patrick Suessmuth, who turned an abandoned school gym into a community centre where kids can race through the halls on inline skates, or play basketball or hopscotch. Or the late Jane Holmes, a parent whose passion for healthier food in the schools resulted in a district-wide healthy food policy for Nova Scotia. I will tell you more about these inspirational people throughout this book. They give me not only hope, but also solid proof that change *is* possible, that we can all play a role in making our communities better.

My friend Ric Young says that all social change happens because a person comes along and speaks a resonant truth to people with an unrealized longing. To me the resonant truth is that our children need to move—they need to be healthy.

We are the generation of superwomen and supermen, and yet even with all the drive in our careers, families and personal goals, we find ourselves coming up just a little bit short. We simply run out of time and energy. The solution is sitting right in front of us, and it isn't a new gadget or organizing technique—it is amazingly simple. In fact, it's child's play. When we give ourselves permission to skip that one music lesson and just hang out in the yard together, go for a walk, connect while shooting some hoops, we take the pressure off. It's child's play.

My oar goes into the water and I pull a stroke; the boat covers a little distance, gains a bit of speed. The first stroke feels heavy, even a little unbalanced. If I stop I'll see that the boat has moved only a little. However, one stroke follows another, and soon the boat gains momentum, cutting through the water with far less heave and ho. I am holding my oars more deftly; by the tenth stroke I find my rhythm and the boat is racing through the water at full speed.

The first strokes that we take in getting our kids active may feel clumsy; we might wonder if we are getting it right. Those first few initiatives we take in our family and community will take effort, and some of that effort will seem awkward and difficult. But if we continue to put our oars in the water, try new initiatives, adapt an idea that is not getting the wanted results, teach a game differently so kids will understand it better, our effort will gain momentum and our boat will start to glide. We might pull only twenty strokes of the race, but our neighbours, our teachers, the young instructor at the recreation centre—they are all pulling too. Together we will win this race for our children's health.

Not everything that can be counted counts,
and not everything that counts can be counted.

ALBERT EINSTEIN

THE VALUE OF PLAY

It's pouring, so the kids and I are inside playing a rather rambunctious game of sledding. The kids dragged the throw off the couch and William is now pulling Kate full speed around the house over our hardwood floors. William is the sled dog and Kate the musher. Kate even knows the right words: she yells "gee, gee" when she wants William to go right, and "haw, haw" for left. They like to take the corners with extra speed, which leads to frequent skids into walls and to the occasional tumble. Now it's my turn to pull William. I get him going at a pretty good speed and of course dump him off the sled at the first turn. We burst into laughter, and listening to his giggles gets me laughing even harder. We start again and I am laughing so hard that I'm having trouble pulling and breathing, so I stop and wait for the laughter to subside before beginning another full-speed tour of the main floor. I delight in my children's uncontained energy, and our joy this evening is palpable. This gets me thinking about joy itself and when we experience it.

When I speak about the value of play, the joy in jumping and running, the thrill of spinning on a swing with a two-year-old in your lap, I am talking about experiences with immense and immeasurable value. If you are looking for facts and figures, they exist, but I doubt that even the best-researched ideas about play and sport would fully articulate the deep value of play to children and communities. How does one measure joy? Joy such as I felt when I held my baby William in my arms for the very first time, or the joy we're experiencing as a family tonight as we fly through the house? I can't tell you exactly how these joyful moments—my very first moments of motherhood, William's giggles, Kate's screams—increase the quality and intensity of my life, but I know these moments have become beacons that guide me in the right direction no matter what else I am doing.

Trying to attach an absolute value to something as abstract as the idea of play is difficult. Why does being chased in fun thrill us? Why will we sleep under the stars on the cold, damp ground just for the slight chance of seeing a shooting star? Why does our entire body relax when we lie on a freshly cut lawn on a hot summer afternoon?

It is because these small moments and simple actions and easy games fill our souls. They delight our senses and sustain us. What is happening to us in those moments is life. We are experiencing life through all our senses, through the momentary connection of our minds, our bodies and our souls. Children know intuitively how to fill their souls. When given the freedom, they live in their bodies and in the natural environment in an integrated way— exploring the backyard ravine, observing water spiders in puddles, changing their make-believe games with the seasons.

Small moments and simple actions and easy games fill our souls.

Andy Anderson, a professor at the University of Toronto, is an expert on the importance of play in child development. "Children delight in the joyful innocence of play," he says. "Through play, we stimulate our senses and experience the grace of our bodies in movement. We nurture our children and we are enriched by the sensational experiences of play."

To a child, the world is full of magic and wonder and possibility, which slowly erode as we hyper-
structure their lives, pressure them to excel, teach
them not to trust anyone. The breakdown of our
neighbourhoods as places where people know and
look out for one another is a real barrier to our children's experiencing this natural integration of their
bodies, mind and souls because it removes the
opportunities for them to run wild through the
neighbourhood or to socialize spontaneously and
creatively, and encourages a subtle yet profound distrust of the people around them. This problem is not
unique to North America. I have spoken to people in
Switzerland and Germany and Mexico who have told
me they are witnessing the same thing—an increasing
disconnection between the mind, the spirit and the
body in children. An internationally respected
Russian rowing coach who has worked in Japan,
America and China told me he sees this as a world-
wide trend. Pointing to his body, he said, "It is as if we
have forgotten that we have a body. Everything lives
here!" In neglecting our physical body, our mind and
spirits suffer too.

Most of us understand that play and sport are
important for children in part because we believe at
an intuitive level that kids and play go together. We've
taken for granted that play would always be a normal

part of our children's experience. But free, unstructured play has all but disappeared from our neighbourhoods and communities. We are just beginning to notice the absence of something we didn't think we would ever have to fight for.

Recently I rowed in an old-timers' race. (It was actually called the Legends Race, but I think most of us succumbed to lactic acid and blisters and decided that we were, quite clearly, old-timers.) It was held on a beautiful rowing course in Lucerne, Switzerland, where I had competed eight times. Every corner of that course held memories, and every "legend" I met reminded me of good times gone by, of the beautiful and difficult things sport has taught me. When we play or compete in sport, we build memories, and these memories—whether of playing softball with our best friends at the neighbourhood park or of competing internationally for Canada—fill our mental diaries. I compare my rowing career to a great love relationship the end of which has not diminished the experience. Memories remain like beloved pictures in my jacket pocket.

When kids play in the streets of our neighbourhood or on the local soccer team, they are creating pictures like these—stories about their childhood that they will remember in some way for the rest of their lives. Television and video games won't create such stories; MSN and chat rooms won't either. First-hand memories are created when our children are fully engaged in life: playing outside, hanging out with their parents or practising with their teammates.

My strongest and most treasured memories of my father are of the times we spent together in the outdoors. Once he took my siblings and me on a cycling trip from Mississauga to Toronto and back one Sunday afternoon, a distance of about fifty kilometres. Such an adventure it was, setting out to cycle to the big city. It was a long way, and we got tired. I remember him pushing my little brother up all the hills and sometimes even coming back down the hill so he could help me through the top bit. Just as I was straining and feeling a whine building up in my throat, my dad's strong hand on the small of my back gave me that much-needed extra push. He would say, "Hey, great going, you're almost at the top," and I would glide effortlessly to the crest.

Our memories of childhood play remind us not only of precious moments with our family, but also of the connections we had to neighbours and friends.

When children play together, particularly in unstructured ways, they learn how to interact with one another. Let's think about that hockey game on a homemade backyard rink: The game was comprised of kids of different ages, and there were no referees or parents telling us to lower our sticks, to score now, to "pass, *pass*, PASS!" We lowered our sticks because our buddies got mad at us, and we had to figure out how to get along with the kids we didn't like. (And sometimes we *were* the kid no one liked.) We were happy to include that weaker player to create even numbers, and if things really got unfair we knew that we needed to work it out or the game could not continue. Playing hockey was so much fun that we didn't want the game to stop, so we learned how to get along with and respect one another—not because our parents told us to, but because respect was the foundation of the game's continuing.

While we were playing, we made new friends, our parents got to know each other and our neighbourhood took on a character of true community. We were invited as families to each other's celebrations; we felt comfortable reaching out when one of us was going through a difficult time, and we started feeling like we were never really alone.

Sport has a transforming effect on children and communities. Here are some things we *can* effectively measure: According to *Investing in Canada: Fostering an Agenda for Citizen and Community Participation*—a public-policy forum report funded by Canadian Heritage—participation in sport, physical activity or other recreation is the single most common way immigrants enter into the mainstream of community life. It is by joining the local soccer or curling leagues that we get outside our homes and connect with one another. For a recent immigrant or for someone who has just moved from one part of the country to another, this connection is essential to feeling part of the community, because it unites people in a common experience. Meeting people through sport takes the intimidation out of living in a brand-new country or brand-new neighbourhood by making us partners, competitors and friends. As I have heard John Furlong, CEO of the 2010 Olympic Games, say many times, sport has a transforming effect on people and community.

I believe most of us long for a strong sense of community. But urban sprawl has led us to live farther from our friends, from our work, from our children's schools and playing fields and parks. Often our families live hundreds of miles or entire continents away. We still have neighbours, but after a day spent commuting, working and ferrying our kids to lessons and practices, we don't have the time (or energy) to really get to know each other. A close friend of mine is a police officer; he tells the story of one robbery that happened in broad daylight—the entire contents of a home were removed, in plain view of the neighbours. When he questioned the people next door, he was told, "I thought something a little odd was going on, but I figured they must be moving or something." After a robbery has occurred in any area, residents always want to know how to protect themselves. "See that door?" my friend says, pointing to a neighbour's house. "Knock on it and say hello."

I don't believe we have suddenly become apathetic about our neighbours and about the well-being and safety of our neighbourhoods. It's just that the mechanics of our lives conspire against lasting connections. We work away from the suburbs, and we work increasingly long hours. In homes with two parents, both are usually working and the children are in after-school care. Families come home together not at three, when school is out, but at five o'clock or later, and often for just enough time to eat a quick meal before heading out to a child's music lesson or sports practice. Having gotten out of the habit of taking time to meet our neighbours, we often don't know how to even begin to meet them. But I have noticed that when someone takes the initiative to reach out and create a block party or a neighbourhood soccer game, everyone goes out of their way to be at the event. We actually *want* to get to know one another—we just need to figure out how.

If we want to create connection within our communities, we must be very purposeful in making it happen. Sometimes it can happen through neighbourhood design, through a strong leader or through a natural disaster (in Victoria, this means a snowstorm). When we have the excuse to connect, we all feel the warmth and support of being part of our community. But we can't rely on such things to do our work for us. When we begin to know our neighbours, to know who lives where, we are more open to the idea of our children being outside in the playgrounds and streets.

Of course, when kids are playing shinny in the cul-de-sac, they are not thinking about strengthening their bones and building their muscle or about making their community a better place; they are playing. And yet physical movement—exercise—is the single most important factor in having a healthy body. It is through movement that our bodies become stronger—not stronger in an "I want to be an Olympic athlete" way, but strong enough to weather the inevitable physical and mental challenges of living. A strong body decreases our risk of disease and injury, and it increases our vibrancy and quality of life.

Exercise leads to stronger bones, healthy lungs, increased endurance and strength. But it also gives us more energy, a positive mindset, an increase in endorphins and more capacity to experience joy. Who wouldn't want these benefits for their kids?

I often hear people say, as they watch children run frantically around the house, "What I wouldn't give for their energy!" As adults, we could have a lot of the energy we see in young children if we committed to a healthier way of being in the world. Playing with our kids not only helps them, it helps us. Kids who are physically active are much more likely to be physically active adults.

When we begin to know our neighbours a little more, to know who lives where, we are more open to the idea of our children being outside in the playgrounds and streets.

And it is natural for children to be physically active. Play is a child's way of exploring the world. A toddler will build a tall castle with blocks and scream with delight when he smashes it down. He is experiencing his ability to have an effect through the simple action of moving his arm. He understands that there are consequences to his actions, that he is a part of this world. All of us who have fought with a young child to contain her in a high chair know that children are designed to move. They are easily angered when a caregiver tries to stop them. Babies who are not given adequate opportunities to move do not develop their motor skills appropriately. Like any other skill, movement has to be experienced and practised to be mastered. Children who do not have good basic motor skills usually become less motivated to move later in childhood and are three times more likely to be sedentary.

As children get older, their need for play doesn't lessen—in fact, it increases—but we tend to devalue its importance. We want our children to excel in academics, to learn an instrument and to become computer literate, and in the process we deprive them of their time for unstructured play and sport. Yet their bodies still need it. And their minds certainly need exercise to release energy so they can stay focused on a task when they need to. There is more research to be done, but studies of children with ADHD show significant improvements in concentration following athletic activity, particularly if it is outdoors. Common sense reminds us of the paradox that we need to move so that we can be still. My parents certainly knew that physical activity was key to us sitting still when we needed to; they insisted we go outside and blow off some steam before Aunt Harriet or whoever came to visit and they would need us to sit down for a while.

It is through movement and play that our children build their joy. I have rarely seen a child who looks unhappy when she is skipping or playing hopscotch. And children who are not supported in their natural desire to move can become disengaged and depressed. Depression is an alarmingly frequent ailment in children now; in North America the prescribing of antidepressants to children has almost doubled over the past five years. Even toddlers are being given psychotropic medication, to treat their hyperactivity—a noxious new response to the terrible twos. Although I am certain that medication is an important part of the treatment of mental illness in some children, my reading and my own experiences working with high-risk youth have shown me that many of the negative indicators of ADHD can be alleviated through adequate activity and a positive social setting.

We want our children to excel in academics, to learn an instrument and to become computer literate, and in the process we deprive them of their time for unstructured play.

In 1994, I became one of the founders of a rowing program for high-risk kids, called Dynamic Opportunities for Youth. Through the support of Dynamic Mutual Funds and the GO Rowing and

Paddling Association of Canada, we put hundreds of kids through an eight-week course focused on building life skills while learning the basics of rowing. In Vancouver, one teenager, built like a Mack truck, boldly strode up to me and declared, "I'm a bad-ass kid." Honestly, I felt a little intimidated, but we stepped into a quadruple scull and I put him into the stroke seat, the lead position. I witnessed his slouchy posture changing immediately, his voice becoming receptive and positive. "Am I doing okay?" he asked. This kid was utterly transformed in the boat. He told me several times that the experience was "wicked."

If we need science to convince us of the cause-and-effect relationship between physical and mental health, top Canadian researchers and academics have already done the research and we should all be reading it. However, we can also trust what we know based on our own experiences and observations, and we need to honour that knowledge by integrating regular, exciting and creative fitness into our families and communities and schools.

Active, healthy children generally feel pride in what their bodies can do, and feel connected to their physical selves. Inactivity in children often leads to low self-esteem, weight issues and even obesity. Being overweight or obese is dangerous for children's health and devastating to their social interactions. Dr.

Gabriela Tymowski, the director of LEAP! (the Learning, Eating, Activity Program) at the University of New Brunswick's pediatric obesity clinic, paints this picture of what life can be like for many overweight and obese children:

> A lot of the kids are bullied and ostracized at school; they can't participate in most activities. For example, we have a little girl who is ten years old and she weighs 217 pounds. She doesn't walk to school; she lives two blocks away and her mother drives her there and back. She doesn't participate in PE because she can't control her body; she falls off her chair, she falls down the stairs, and each time something like that happens it has an impact on her self-esteem so she doesn't want to move. It's safest for her to be sitting somewhere and not moving . . . She's not a "normal" child in the school—she's "different," and she's only ten years old . . . Kids do tell me, the older ones, about how unhappy they are, how sad they are all the time, how miserable they feel—and unfortunately, a number of them turn to eating for solace and tend to barricade themselves in their rooms at home.

On the other hand, involvement in play and sports can have a positive effect on children's self-esteem. Kids who play sports in their teen years are far less likely to smoke or use drugs. This is not just because they are busy, but because when we use our bodies to run and jump and play, we have a deeper respect for our physical selves.

Last weekend, I went with my kids to a friend's house, on a five-acre property. There, the parents were letting their children grow up playing outside. My kids spent the next five hours swinging from a rope ladder, playing hide and seek and finding bugs in a tiny stream at the edge of the property. These young people who had never met each other began interacting instantly, using their imaginations to make up games. When children play together, particularly outside, they rely upon their imaginations: the water hose gets turned on and a dam is built; blankets get dragged outside and a fort is made. Kids move from one activity to another, living delightfully in the world of make-believe. When I came outside to see how my kids were doing, I sat down on a log near where they were playing. "You are sitting on our life raft!" one of the boys scolded me.

With all this emphasis on play, I don't want you to think I'm downplaying the value of organized sport (though it feels less endangered). When kids play an organized sport, they have an opportunity to create a meaningful relationship with adults other than their parents. Young people often turn to their coaches for leadership and advice; they respect their opinions and cherish their guidance. As parents, we need to watch over these relationships, but a healthy relationship with a good coach can really make a difference in a child's life. It is important that kids know that adults care about them, and sometimes it is very important that children have an adult to talk to who isn't a parent. My coaches counselled me on what university to attend, how to communicate with my parents and even what to wear to the high school prom.

Working with Seppo Peuhkurinen, my running coach when I was twelve, was my first significant relationship with an adult outside my family. He helped me set goals and understand my abilities. He cared about me. Now, I look back and realize how extraordinary it was that he shared his time with so many children and young adults, even when he had his own kids to raise.

Seppo talked to me about having dreams and setting goals. I remember sitting down with him at the beginning of the track season and deciding on a specific time (2 minutes 16 seconds) to aim for in the 800-metre. It was my first experience in setting goals.

He would ask me to actually write down what I wanted to achieve. Part of me thought the process was a bit hokey, but today I am deeply grateful for the approach he taught me. Playing sport opened up a new world for me, where there were dreams and goals and challenges. Suddenly, I not only had a plan for my sport performance, but began to plan and dream for my life.

From sport, children can learn to be responsible for their own performances, on the playing field and in life.

Of course, we know, as adults, that our dreams change, and that regardless of our desire and hard work, sometimes our efforts don't yield the desired results. Sport teaches this too—to be gracious in winning because losing is inevitable. In my experience, every true champion has an enormous desire to win, but also this graciousness: the humility to know that winning is sweet yet temporal.

Among the attitudes sports taught me are optimism, determination, a respect for fair play, teamwork, and perhaps the most valuable lesson: to be honest with myself. When I competed, I was the only one who really knew how any given race had unfolded. I could always find excuses for a bad performance, but it was only through honesty that I could see my shortcomings and work through them.

It has helped me know when I have not worked hard enough, when I have made the error of underestimating a task or a competition; it holds me accountable for my successes and my setbacks. Just as a great athlete first turns to himself to find the answer to why the game did not go his way, so a complete person asks himself what he needs to learn, what he can do better when confronted by an event that did not unfold the way he imagined. This approach has helped me recover from small mishaps, such as a poor audience reaction to a new presentation, and from life-changing crises, such as the end of my marriage. From sport, children can learn to be responsible for their own performances, on the playing field and in life.

In the end, my playing field included the whole world. Those exotic-sounding names were merely places on a map before I began to travel internationally in the sport of rowing. I assumed that people from different countries were different from me, that they would have different motivations and significantly different attitudes. At the world championships in Germany, in 1983, I waited for the weigh scales behind an enormously muscular Russian rower. She weighed in at 220 pounds, and as she stepped off the scales I stood back in awe. She was superhuman. I spent the next couple of days at the regatta simply in fear of all the powerful women who were there to compete. Two days later, during a qualifying round, a girl in the Russian boat caught a crab—put her blade in the water at the wrong angle, causing it to dive deeply into the water and stop the boat. The team still managed to qualify, but after the race I saw the girl from the weigh scales, that superhuman, in tears of frustration. Her coach came up to her and gave her a hug, and she suddenly became a little more human in my eyes. Competing with athletes from different cultures and countries often challenged my preconceived ideas.

> In order to win the game for their team, they have to see past their differences—they have to stop looking at each other as enemies and pass the ball.

Playing sport breaks through religious, cultural and political differences. This can be seen in a program called Playing for Peace, which brings Palestinian and Israeli children together on the basketball court. The children learn to see their teammates and competition as just that: teammates and competition. In order to win the game for their team, they have to see past their differences—they have to stop looking at each other as enemies and pass the ball. Sport can be a powerful way of seeing beyond our prejudices. Playing for Peace also works with Protestant and Catholic kids in Ireland to create peaceful relationships out of antagonistic and potentially dangerous ones. It's hard to hate someone who fed you the ball for your winning layup; it's almost impossible to ignore someone on the street who was billeted with you for a tournament.

In 1990 I met Juri Jaansen, a successful sculler from Yugoslavia, and we ended up attending several functions together. Whenever somebody would introduce Juri as the sculler from Yugoslavia, Juri would interrupt and say adamantly, "No, I am from Slovenia!" He would begin to explain the politics of that region, and I remember his passion for his country, the freedom it represented to him and his need to help others understand. I thought to myself at the time, "I ought to know about this—this is important." As an athlete at the top of my game, I lived from practice to practice with little awareness of politics outside my sport. Yet Juri made me aware that these new countries emerging rapidly in Europe had been hard won. They weren't just new borders for the West to learn, but liberation for many, many people.

The fall of the Berlin Wall is something that is etched in my mind. In November 1990, at the world championships, rowers from West and East Germany competed against each other for the last time. After the races, you could see athletes from both countries hugging each other and welcoming one another as teammates. It was sad to see the East Germans take their uniforms off, but also inspiring and moving to see the support and good wishes for the Germans being spread throughout the regatta by all of the competitors.

Seeing the world through sport is an exceptional and unusual benefit to competing; however, this understanding of one another works the same way in our neighbourhoods and local leagues. Play brings us together and moves us beyond our preconceived notions. Play asks us to get along, to work within the boundaries of fair play and to respect one another. Respect for each other in our communities—and for the community that is the world—is the foundation of good citizenship and healthy relations.

The health of our communities begins with the health of each one of us. Being healthy in body, mind and spirit is what we wish for every child. Health, so they can move into adulthood ready to tackle the opportunities and challenges of life. Health, so their bodies are strong, their minds are clear and their spirits are buoyant. Health, because we want them to understand the relationship between their moods and their bodies, to know they can change their inner dialogues with some yoga or some fresh air. Health, because we want them to recognize their bodies, not as something that makes them feel tired or that they are ashamed of, but as the temple for their minds, their ideas, their dreams. Play is a vital component to good mental health, particularly in children, so we must never forget that children need to play to be healthy. Their minds need it, their bodies crave it and their spirits are elevated by it.

The greatest value of sport is the joy it brings us, and this joy is not limited to kids. We all know how much fun it is to play with our kids. Playing lets us get outside our heads, outside our daily stresses, outside our jobs. And for our kids it is a time to de-stress about school or to get space away from friendships that are confusing or unhealthy. It is a place where we can all just be. Moving our bodies energizes us; it releases endorphins and fosters joy, and joy ought never to be sidelined in what we do. Joy fosters hope, and hope is everything. Let's never lose sight that it is this—something we can't measure and can barely articulate—that is the most important part of playing, the most important part of childhood. In fact, let's all take a moment to do something joyful with our kids right now. I'm always up for another round of house-sledding.

"You are the sum of the decisions you make."
Olympic gold medallist Simon Whitfield

THE BAD NEWS

In a time when parents are focused more than ever before on doing the right thing for their kids, it is difficult to grasp how we have gone so wrong. What we hear in the news about the health of our children sends us reeling: they are not getting enough exercise to grow and develop optimally; almost 40% of our children are overweight; and Type II diabetes—previously unheard of in children—is escalating to frightening proportions. Despite the enormous emphasis we put on providing absolutely every opportunity for our children, somehow we are failing in our most fundamental responsibility: to foster their physical health and well-being.

Dropping the Ball: Canada's Report Card on Physical Activity for Children and Youth (2005), based on research conducted by Active Healthy Kids Canada, an association that promotes physical activity opportunities for all Canadian children and youth, gave us a failing grade. Our schools scored an F, our community environment a C and our family activity levels a D. This is not a report card

Numerous health experts believe that we will be the first generation to live longer than our children.

parents would welcome if their child brought it home. When you know your child can do better, you do whatever you can to help him or her. Well, this is *our* report card, and it's telling us we can all do better for our kids and families and communities. This report card should be our call to action.

We are bewildered as parents, as physicians, as a society: Where and how have we gone so wrong? Our children, as a whole, are not healthy. Their quality of life has been severely compromised by inactivity. Numerous health experts believe that we will be the first generation to live longer than our children. Our children are being deprived of full lives, not just in terms of the activities they can do, but also in terms of their self-esteem, their energy, their joy for life. Some will never know what it feels like to be healthy. We are all struggling to grasp how we got here, and many of us hardly know where to begin to turn this terrible tide. But we must be prepared to take a look at our values and parenting methods to see where our own personal responsibility lies. We cannot afford to spend precious energy pointing fingers; we need to take action.

I believe every parent's desire is for their child to have a real childhood. A childhood filled with the joy of just playing.

Let's look at the facts—the statistics and stories that paint the picture of our children's health today. These facts are bleak, yes—they are frightening, they are undeniable—but their function is not to paralyze and overwhelm us. Facts are invaluable because they show us where we once were and where we are now; they also give us direction on where to go and help us develop a plan to get there. Using facts this way is an approach I call "realistic optimism." Realistic optimism is built on belief and faith: belief that change is possible and faith that no matter how big the gap appears, we can surmount it.

The facts we have now are revealing the world our children live in, a world we barely recognize, a world we are responsible for creating.

Half of children in North America do not get enough physical activity for optimal growth and development. "Optimal development" refers to the full potential of both the physical and the mental growth of our children. To grow optimally means they are exhausted at the end of the day from using their bodies and feeling the wind and weather on their faces—not because they are crashing from a sugar and junk-food high, or because they are burdened with heavy, sluggish bodies, or because computer games or the TV has burned them out. It means they are tired from being kids all day! I believe every parent's desire is for their child to have a real childhood. A childhood filled with the joy of just playing. This belief is the inspiration for this book. And I believe we care enough to take action. It is up to each of us to help create a better world for our kids.

Dr. Heather McKay, an associate professor in the Faculty of Medicine at UBC, has been working in the area of bone health for most of her career. She was the lead researcher of the Action Schools! BC project, based on the widely researched and supported idea that the antecedents of almost all chronic diseases are present in childhood. Dr. McKay's research looks at intervening during childhood to positively affect children's health, physical activity and nutrition.

Until a few years ago, we had very little idea of how a healthy skeleton develops. Dr. McKay led a seven-year trial that studied how children accrue bone and how they develop their skeletons. "We learned that 23% of our adult skeleton is formed in two years during a very crucial time in adolescence," says Dr. McKay. "Obviously this led to the question of what kids are doing in adolescence—usually they are doing all the wrong things. Today we have a natural experiment whereby we are introducing physical *inactivity* into children's lives. What happens when that happens?"

There is a window, starting in the year following the greatest growth spurt (which is later for boys), when the skeleton is sensitive to exercise. No wonder their appetites skyrocket! During that time, it is critical that children's growing bones are regularly stressed or loaded through physical activity. As Dr. McKay explains, it is a once-in-a-lifetime opportunity: "If you withdraw that from an adolescent, you will never again have the same opportunity to reach optimal bone strength." Dr. McKay's studies give us a clear understanding of the necessity of exercise during these critical years. I was amazed to learn that the skeleton actually resorbs itself if it is not used enough. If your bones do not get stimulus through loading, your body gets the message that it doesn't need that bone and begins to resorb it. This resorption happens ten times faster during childhood.

Dr. McKay stresses the importance of acting on this research now: "I think we are going to see a huge implication for this population of children when they reach adulthood. We haven't seen the worst of it yet. This is why governments are paying attention; we can't wait until 40% of the population are sustaining fragility fractures." Corporations are beginning to pay attention, too, because they can no longer afford to ignore the poor health of this generation. These unfit kids will be their employees of tomorrow, and many companies already have a big problem, spending more on health care than they do on their product.

In addition to building strong adult skeletons, children need to exercise their lungs at this age, as this is when we develop much of our adult lung capacity. In the area of cardiovascular fitness, children are doing significantly less well than they were twenty years ago. Another study measured the cardiovascular endurance of kids today. It found that cardiovascular endurance is on average 30% lower than in 1980. Those of us who coach sports or play actively with children on a regular basis know there are a startling number of kids who can't run around the track once, and who at the tender age of six already feel encumbered by their bodies.

According to the health report card, our children are among the most inactive and most overweight in the world. The obesity rate of Canadian boys between the ages of eight and twelve appears to be almost as high as it is in the US, where it is arguably the highest in the world. This statistic is shocking; we are beginning to see the harsh health consequences of our children's lifestyle.

People seem to have forgotten that kids need fresh air and exercise, and lots of it.

When I had dinner with a group of nurses in Edmonton, they told me about the number of bypass surgeries they are seeing for people in their twenties, something that rarely happened a decade ago. These twenty-somethings are the product of an inactive, nutritionally deficient era. Similarly, Dr. Andrew Pipe talks about studies that identify hardening of the arteries in children as young as four. When I visited him at the University of Ottawa Heart Institute, he showed me a graph charting two things: the physical activity levels of children, which have been steadily declining over the past fifteen years, and the number of overweight and obese children, which has been rising at the same rate. It certainly got my attention.

Professor Mark Tremblay, chair of Active Healthy Kids Canada, is an advocate and top researcher in the area of physical activity and kids. In an article for the *National Post*, commenting on the results of the report card, his frustration with the current state of children's health came through loud and clear: "These problems have been predictable for some time ... It seems that things need to get very, very bad before we start paying attention to them." How bad are we willing to let things get?

To fully understand the impact of our children's inactive lifestyle, we must also consider their emotional and mental health. People seem to have forgotten that kids need fresh air and exercise, and lots of it. Fresh air is a proven component in good mental health and is recommended by counsellors and psychiatrists as an antidote to mental illness.

The children who now make up our statistics on obesity are part of a generation that has not been given adequate opportunities to be active—not by their families, not by their schools, not by their communities. Canadian thirteen-year-old girls spend on average more than three hours each day chatting on MSN and cruising the World Wide Web. Although 68% of kids play sports, only 50% of the lowest-income kids in this country play sports (as compared to almost 80% of the highest-income kids). This means that 32% of kids overall don't play sports, and that's too many inactive children. Maybe 50% of the lowest-income kids playing sports is better than nothing, but we as a society should not accept that thousands of children are missing the opportunity of a lifetime due to circumstances beyond their control.

We are struggling on a personal level, but our institutions are letting us down too. In elementary schools, we have generalist teachers teaching physical education with little or no training and inadequate support. Who can blame teachers for not enthusing about PE when they are not properly equipped to teach this subject to the standard of excellence

The behaviour of our kids—their patterns of spending their time watching videos, being inactive at recess and not walking to school are not long-term patterns, nor long-standing ways of living; they have occurred over the last generation.

they bring to other subjects? Funding cuts and a narrow focus on academic excellence in core subjects like science, math and reading have reduced the richness of the school experience for our children. But recent studies illustrate that a robust physical activity program—including PE, schoolyard games and active classrooms—helps create a positive attitude toward school. Before my son asks to stay home when he is not feeling well, he always asks if it is a gym day.

Studies show that our children spend 50% less time outdoors than they did twenty years ago. Fifty percent! Why is this happening? As Steve Friesen, a passionate PE teacher from Guelph, Ontario, says, "Kids don't want to feel sad, they don't want to be fat, and they aren't lazy." It is just too easy for us to say that kids today are lazy, that kids today eat junk, that kids today don't want to be outdoors. They are *our* kids, and we have played a major role in forming their approach to life, to the choices they are making today. We have either forgotten or ignored our responsibility for teaching our children the basic yet critical elements of feeling good and being healthy.

These changes in our kids' activity levels, outdoor time and obesity rate have happened over the past fifteen years, a relatively short time span. The behaviour of our kids—their patterns of spending their time watching videos, being inactive at recess and not walking to school—are not long-term patterns, nor long-standing ways of living; they have occurred over the last generation, and it is up to us to admit that what we are doing is not good enough.

When you walk the streets in the evening, you rarely see families playing outside together, riding their bikes or playing a game of soccer. Of course, as parents we are more exhausted than ever before, so it's hard to imagine how we can help our kids to become more active. Many parents are both working outside the home, coming home exhausted and then hustling to take their kids to an activity. Also, many parents don't feel qualified to teach their kids how to throw a baseball or kick a soccer ball—we have given our role to the "experts," believing that if our kids don't receive proper instruction, they will not realize their full potential. But as a friend and single father of three confided to me, "Sometimes I think the driving, the rushing is unsustainable. I love participating in my kids' activities, but I also wonder, is all this rushing around the best way to live in families?"

As kids get older, they want to play on teams, to be part of a social group. That's natural and healthy, but all kids—both young and old—need to have a broader experience of being active. Any involvement in sports should be enhanced with some neighbourhood games, some fun time spent with parents. Casual, unstructured playing was how most of our bodies became strong and healthy and how many of us developed a lifelong appreciation of exercise. Most Olympic athletes I know, myself included, gained their foundation in a casual and unstructured way.* I was inducted into Canada's

---

*I began rowing at seventeen, but the physical foundation I had acquired from unstructured play helped me make the Olympic team after only two years of rowing.

Sports Hall of Fame the same year as Mario Lemieux, and I still remember his account of playing ball hockey in the front hall of his family's home when it was too cold to go outside. I have this image of three brothers whacking their sticks on the drywall, their mother half glad the kids were occupied so she could prepare dinner and half horrified at the destruction they were probably causing.

When we stop rushing around, there are the screens—television, computer games, MSN, Xbox—all of them competing ferociously for our children's time and attention. Today, creating video and computer games for children is a multi-million-dollar, business and companies want their games to be engrossing and exciting. The sophistication and creativity in these games capture our children's attention and steal their time. Almost a quarter of our kids use the computer more than three hours a day. Add television to this equation and it becomes staggering. A full third of Canadian kids watch more than four hours of television each weeknight, and half our kids watch more than four hours each weekend night. A startling number of little kids aged two to eight have televisions in their bedrooms—65% of kids over eight.

As parents, we need to pay attention to the amount of time our children are spending being passive, not moving. Mark Tremblay warns that even a great exercise session does not replace twenty-three of sloth-like behaviour.

"Depending on what you read," says Dr. Heather McKay, "you see stats that show a 15 to 20% increase in childhood obesity over the last fifteen years. Why? Who are these kids who would not have been in this statistic fifteen years ago? These are the ones that can go either way; these are the ones you and I are probably talking about. Success in this regard is about access, opportunity and modelling. You will always have kids who are going to be active no matter what, and those who will be inactive no matter what you do. It's the people in the middle we can most affect."

When it comes to our kids, too often what we do, we do without intention. Twenty years ago, we played without intention—not to be healthy and well, but simply because that is how children were in the world. Today we allow our kids to play without intention, but the time is spent on video games, chatting on MSN, sitting passively in front of the television. As parents we must become aware and intentional about how our kids are spending their time. We must begin to understand that *how* they spend their time is of paramount importance to their mental, physical and social well-being. We need to create safe places for kids to gather and then they will play.

We also need to recognize our role in teaching our children to make nutritious choices when they eat. At parties, I've often seen the healthy foods like fish, steamed vegetables and organic cheese offered to the adults, while the kids are given chicken nuggets and fries or a simple bowl of pasta with no vegetables or meat. We make so many assumptions about what kids want to eat. Most of us enjoy french fries, pizza and ice cream because the fat and sugar in those foods make them tasty. As adults, we try to edit our choices, knowing we can have fries once a week but not every day, knowing that chocolate cake is fine for the weekend but not for dessert every night. Most of us also acknowledge that certain foods just don't make us feel good. Consuming a cola and fries an hour before a run just doesn't feel as good as eating a piece of fruit or a light meal. And we know that eating too much bread and butter affects our waistline. So why don't we pay the same attention to what our children are eating—not only during the dinners we prepare, but all day? I hear myself say, "Oh, it's just once in a while" as I hand my kids a fat-laden muffin because I didn't take the time to prepare a healthy snack. But once in a while can so easily become far too often. We need to

We need to create safe places for kids to gather and then they will play.

be vigilant, to pass on this learning to our kids, first through example and then through knowledge.

This is the chapter of bad news. Our kids are unwell, and we need to find the strength and energy to take action. Our kids need us to find a way to exist in communities differently, to create opportunities in our neighbourhoods, in our backyards and in our parks for kids to play. We must look at our families and become conscious of the choices we make about how we live as family units. Our children demand that we show a greater vigilance—not just in keeping them safe, but in keeping them healthy.

We need to find the courage. We must resist becoming overwhelmed by the negatives of where we are. The proof that change is possible is all around us, and it is in the stories you will read in the following chapters. The people and programs in these stories give us all the proof that we need: change is not only possible, it is happening, and it is the only option. There are all sorts of people like you and me who have said, "This is simply not good enough for our children." We must do better on behalf of our kids; we can make their world a healthier, better place.

"I want to be a fit."

KYLIE, AGE 7

"I like Play in the Park, because we get to beat the parents, and then I get to walk home with my dad."

ROBERT, AGE 8

FAMILY PLAY

So where do we start? We start at home. Peers are important, and teachers and coaches are part of the equation, but it is the family that plays the primary role in shaping the values and attitudes of our children. Parenting experts, researchers and social scientists emphasize it over and over again: the parent–child relationship is the most important relationship a person will have in his or her lifetime.

This is great if you think you're doing everything perfectly. However, if you're like me, this responsibility might make you feel a little nervous. Imperfect parent that I am, I stubbed my toe on the corner of my bed last night and shouted, "Damn!" at the top of my lungs in pain and frustration. Last week, overwrought with my own day (and, okay, a little hormonal), when my daughter decided to have a little meltdown, I melted down right alongside her. Sometimes we aren't proud of our behaviour, but it is comforting to know that our kids are actually taking in some of the positive things we do and say.

> Because children *do* observe how we live our lives, our rules and guidance have a tremendous impact on the choices they make in theirs.

When I do yoga, my son often sits down on the floor beside me and imitates the frog position. "Look, Mommy, I can do it!" he calls to me. My little girl studies my face in the mirror as I put on my lipstick and then asks if she may try. I hear echoes of my influence in their little voices. "No, I am concentrating," Kate chides William when he interrupts her intent colouring. "Goldfish are a once-in-a-while food," William tells Kate as we navigate the cracker aisle of our local grocer. (And children draw their own conclusions from actions and events we *don't* explain to them. The mysterious disappearance of our family's pet rabbits left me speechless. William concluded that Princess and Curious were happy because they were free to meet other bunnies! I am sure the rabbit population in our neighbourhood is thankful for that.) Kate spent the summer watching me write this book, and she regularly tells her friends she is going to write a book soon. In fact, she recently presented me with the first chapter of *Adventure Princess Has a Party*. Children learn from what their parents do and say, and from how they respond to situations. They study us to try to understand the world around them.

Because children *do* observe how we live our lives, our rules and our guidance have a tremendous impact on the choices they make in theirs. It is not enough to love our children—it is not nearly enough. We must set an example and truly think about what they are learning from their family environments. As Barbara Coloroso has put it, we must create environments that give them "the gift of inner discipline." When I ask Kate to try to swim across the pool one more time, she is learning that doing something fun takes an initial effort. She tries all afternoon, first grabbing the ledge of the pool as she swims the entire length, then letting go for a few strokes before frantically grabbing the ledge again. I slip into the pool beside her, encouraging her, reassuring her, and she swims the entire length. She shouts, "I did it, I did it!" as she touches the wall of the deep end. When William slams down his pencil in frustration over his math book, I find a quiet place we can work together and insist that we finish the page. I know he is frustrated by his math homework, but I also know that when he finishes it he will feel a tiny spark of accomplishment. Whether we are conscious of it or not, we are always teaching our kids through example and through the guidance, limits and consequences we provide in our family environments.

Spending time together as a family is a special part of childhood for kids and their parents. Holding our babies, throwing a ball in the backyard with our little boys, teaching our little girls to ride a bicycle— these are the moments we dream about before having children. And when our children arrive, we happily discover that they want to be with us too. A young toddler cries when his mother leaves the room; a two-year-old screams, "Daddy, Daddy!" when her father arrives home at night. When given the opportunity to kick a ball in the backyard with Mom or Dad or to fly a kite in the park with Auntie Shelagh, most kids will delight in the opportunity to be with family. I love these times, when I allow the world to stop and just live in the moment with my children. When I escape my busy life to spend fifteen minutes outside teaching my daughter to skip, I know it is time well spent. Kate loves these one-on-one playtimes with her mommy, and we are building a bond by doing something as simple as skipping rope together. I try to have a moment like this with each of my children once a day.

Although I am sad to admit it, sometimes being together doesn't occur until late at night. When the phone has stopped ringing and the house is peaceful, the three of us lie in my king-size bed and tell the "story of the day," a ritual we look forward to, in which we each get the chance to share something that happened to us.

Playing with my children forces me to push aside my own busyness and distracted head. Sometimes it is only twenty minutes of uninterrupted play, but how precious these minutes are! And when we ride our bikes with our kids or play a game of four-square in the cul-de-sac, our kids are developing their attitudes about physical play and what it means to be a family.

Yes, we are busy, but we have to keep things in perspective, and avoid falling into what I call the "superparent syndrome." I suspect most women over sixty are thinking it, watching the way we are raising our kids, observing the comings and goings of the young families in the neighbourhood—they are thinking, "You're crazy!" In fact, Ellie Donahue, a sixty-plus mom and grandma from Pender Island was bold enough to say it out loud: "You girls are crazy. You drive all over town taking your kids to this and that lesson, you jump up to entertain them every time they look bored. Why don't you just sit down together and have a coffee? The kids will be fine!" My own mother has said it to me so many times. "Just relax."

A coffee? I think for many women the idea of having a coffee with a girlfriend while the kids play contently is a distant fantasy. We are so busy running from one commitment to the next that we rarely have the empty space in our day to contemplate an impromptu meeting with neighbours and friends. Even if we had the time, it would be unlikely that we would find a neighbour home, because she is probably working or busy chauffeuring one of her little ones to dance or an older child to tutoring.

My first September with both kids in school was a bit of a shock. I guess I thought that once the kids were in school, life would become less demanding. Then came the notices from school, the special plays and assemblies, a club that needs a parent's help, the reading and homework time needed between parent and child. I am thrilled that my kids go to a school that engages them in so much; however, I sometimes feel as if I am just not keeping up with their own busy schedules and mine. My calendar is blocked solid every day with their lessons and appointments, my meeting times and conference calls, and the special events and

practices we attend together. Worst of all is my fear—
my fear of forgetting an important item on the piano-
practice schedule, my fear of losing library books to the
chaos of my home, my fear of forgetting that I am driving for today's field trip.

And then the unspoken one: the fear of not being a good parent.

We are so busy going from one commitment to the next that we rarely have the empty space in our day to contemplate an impromptu meeting with neighbours and friends.

I have girlfriends who stay home full-
time with their kids, others who work a
twenty-hour week, and others who have demanding full-time careers. What
we have in common is guilt. I work full-time and
travel quite a bit, constantly worrying about missing
Remembrance Day assemblies, a dance recital, my
daughter's first loose tooth. My assistant, Laurie,
works half-time and worries about work when she is
with her kids and about her kids when she is at work.
Another friend is home part-time; she worries she is
not contributing financially to the family and believes
she should be doing everything perfectly because,
after all, she is at home all day. And all of us secretly
believe that another woman might have worked out a
better equation than we have.

On a girls' weekend away, a close friend of mine made a comment about children who have nannies. She observed that children who live in homes with nannies tend to be less independent and sometimes speak to babysitters and nannies with disrespect. She then gave an example: at a recent outing at the BMX track, my daughter, Kate, had asked our nanny to get her helmet. My friend observed that she was perfectly capable of getting it on her own but clearly expected somebody else to do it. My friend meant well, and she confirmed something I was already seeing in my children. But what surprised me was my reaction: sitting in the back seat of the car on the way home, I found myself feeling really upset. When another girlfriend asked if I was okay, I started to cry.

Criticism of our kids cuts us to the quick. I remember taking my son, William, home from the hospital, all wrinkled and new, and thinking, I'm never going to let anything happen to you. I whispered in his tiny ear, "Mommy is going to take such good care of you." But no sooner had I said it than I started making mistakes, like putting the wrong kind of diaper cream on, which made his bum a flaming red; like bringing him to a remote island hours after his first booster shot and holding him, aghast, as he went limp and pale in my arms; like meeting his midnight demand for feeding with resentful growls of exhaustion. The euphoria of his birth crashed into the inevitable paradoxes of mothering. You love them so much, but at times you feel like running away from them. You wouldn't let a teacher or coach yell at them, yet you find yourself shouting at the top of your lungs, "Go to bed!" or something worse.

At a dinner party recently, I admitted to feeling absolute rage when my son takes out his homework anxieties on me. I have to leave the room, because I feel so frustrated and attacked as he tells me, "I know!" and "Leave me alone!" and "It's your fault!"—all in the same sentence. My girlfriend exclaimed, "When I practise piano with my son and he whines, 'I don't want to practise' for the fifth time that day, I feel like shaking him—I get so mad I have to leave the room or I'm afraid I will yell at him, 'You little spoiled brat—just practise!'" Out came other stories of mother rage, but somehow expressing something that probably startles us all makes us feel more capable of working through these powerful emotions. It's not all cute little baby clothes and "I love you, Mommy" moments. I am so grateful to have a group of friends who aren't afraid to be real, who give each other permission to talk about the underbelly of the parenting experience.

But what about the parents who don't have a circle of people they can do this kind of sharing with? The other parents who are overwhelmed with rage, exhaustion and resentment while feeling deep love and commitment to their children? Perhaps by showing the courage to be real about our shortcomings and our conflicting experiences in parenting, we alleviate a tiny bit of that unrealistic expectation we all live with.

We have what it takes—we really do: we can get better, we can learn more; we are fully capable of being great parents.

We don't get a lot of positive reinforcement in the job of parenting. There is no coach saying "good job" when we make a tough call. There is often nobody in our life who tells us we have done right by denying our kids a privilege, or by talking to them rather than screaming at them. Even if we are getting some of that great coaching from our partners and our own parents, we are constantly assaulted with what we "must do" next: the "proper" way to talk to our kids, the "proper" way to teach our kids to throw a ball, the "proper" way to discipline inappropriate behaviour. Keeping up is exhausting and sometimes just plain discouraging. I have taken a ten-week parenting course by local counsellor Allison Rees that I would recommend to all parents. I read Barbara Coloroso's *Kids Are Worth It* with the kind of fervour appropriate to a holy text. But we need to balance this plethora of information and great guidance with our own common sense and with something even more important: confidence. We have what it takes—we really do: we can get better, we can learn more; we are fully capable of being great parents. When we have that kind of confidence, an observation about our child can feel less personal and we can be objective about its accuracy. We can take a parenting course and feel inspired rather than overwhelmed.

Overwhelmed. There is a word most parents can relate to. *Isolated* is another. Parenting can be a disturbingly isolating experience for many people. Many parents believe their challenges are unique, and they are not comfortable turning to others for support. But help is out there. Parenting workshops and support groups help people realize that although the details of the problems may be different, the issue is usually the same right across the board. Parents discover that they all have had similar experiences, and as a group they can problem-solve together; they realize they are not alone. As an athlete, I worked with coaches who understood the power of encouragement. My coach Mike Spracklen always took the time to give me positive comments about my rowing and always asked me how I perceived the workout and my technique before offering any feedback on what I could do better. He anchored his criticism in plenty of positive observations and generous praise. It might sound Pollyannaish, but I believe praise and positive observations work—they assist us in letting down our guard and making space for that important feedback that makes us better. I have read that the ideal ratio of encouragement is 5 to 1; most of us give and receive this ratio in opposite proportions.

When a girlfriend takes a moment to tell me that I am doing a great job and that she admires how I combine work and family, when my dad comments on the beautiful handwriting of my five-year-old, I feel more capable as a parent. I must remember to send more positive encouragement to the people in my life—to the neighbour who seems tired and overwhelmed, to the friend going through a divorce and learning to cope with split parenting. I tried it on this morning at my child's school. I mentioned to a mom at the school that I was impressed by how her son had opened the door for a smaller child. I told another what great energy she had with her kids. Maybe these comments will cast some rays of white and healing light into our beat-up parental psyches.

Not long ago I asked a friend how she was managing her successful real estate career with two small children, and she burst into tears: "I feel like I am missing all the important stuff." Another friend, who stays home with her two- and four-year-olds shared with me how she visualized herself as this person who was slowly disappearing into shadow form. "Pretty soon, I'll forget who I am," she laughed wryly.

So maybe we've got to admit this parenting stuff is pretty tough. There isn't a perfect balance, and there isn't a right and wrong way of doing things. If we can stop assuming others are judging us, maybe we can reinvest that energy in support-ing each other. On one day when I got off the airplane and went straight to the school to pick up my children, another mother commented on how empa-thetic my daughter had been when her little boy fell in the playground. Her words of praise for my little girl almost made me cry. I make a conscious effort to tell my ex-husband at every opportunity what a great dad he is; I know my words are true, and they make him even better. And that's the thing: kind words directed at another make us better.

I can stand in the middle of my vibrant, full and wonderful life and feel utterly and completely overwhelmed by the sheer pace of it.

Like so many parents, sometimes I am just hanging on. I can stand in the middle of my vibrant, full and wonderful life and feel utterly and completely over-whelmed by the sheer pace of it. To all the parents out there whose lives are different from mine, who may not have a nanny or even the cash to hire a babysitter, I applaud you. To the moms who work and drop off their little babies at daycare by 7:30 a.m. so that you can make it to work on time, I can only imagine the fatigue and stress you feel. My girlfriend had her first baby at twenty-two while her husband was still in grad school and she was finishing a degree in communications. While I was out rowing at 6:30 a.m. on a lake in Victoria, she was bundling up baby Kira to brave the sub-zero Winnipeg temperatures and drop her at daycare. Every night, she'd collect Kira at 6:00 p.m., exhausted by a full day of work and school. They would go home and do it all over the next day. This is life for many parents, and I am deeply respectful of the patience and endurance they exhibit in order to be good parents to their little ones.

Parenting is exhausting. It makes us cry; it can make us feel overwhelmed and inadequate. I believe we need to find ways to support one another through these years, to share what is working rather than focusing on where we feel we are inadequate. The best thing we can do for ourselves is to stop comparing, stop trying to be perfect, stop exhausting ourselves trying to provide every opportunity for our kids. We need to be real with them, to spend time with them and let go of some of the little details that overwhelm us.

I think a lot of us hold this image of what an

"ideal" parent is. This person bakes her Thanksgiving cake two days ahead and then decorates it with little orange and red turkeys. Her child has a gym bag that was made on the family sewing machine, eats home-made cookies and is patiently helped with his reading and homework each and every night. This couldn't be more different than my life of spelling tests given on the way to school, reading done with a child while I am falling asleep, and harried cries of "hurry up, hurry up" permeating the house both morning and night.

Last week I made a beautiful apple crisp for Kate's Thanksgiving lunch at school but forgot to tell my family it was for Kate's party. When I went to pack it, I was horrified to see that a big chunk was missing. Too late to bring something else, Kate arrived at school with a half-eaten dish.

We all have a little gremlin who sits on our shoulder and talks to us about ourselves and our abilities. He is not very nice. He doesn't tell us how great we are, that we are doing a fantastic job, that our dreams are worthwhile. He is the voice of fear and doubt. My gremlin is a skeptical and humourless man. He questions my judgment, thinks my dreams are audacious, and always asks who do I think I am to take this risk, to want to do things differently. He is the guy who tells me I am never enough. But lately I have refused to pay him much heed. My gremlin is not going to help me live a better life; the fear and doubt do not make me a better parent. Maybe my gremlin is never going to go away, but I no longer believe he is going to give me an empowering perspective on my life. Perhaps the best thing we can do is become more confident parents.

I think that was what my mother was trying to say to me when she read a piece I had written for an anthology of essays on parenting, in which, again, I mused on the challenges of motherhood. "Silken, you are driving yourself—nuts. You are doing a great job." And most of us are—most of us are doing a great job. I think we just have to give ourselves permission to lighten up, to take time to play with our kids and to unload some activities so that we can just be.

We need to give ourselves permission to do less so we can do more. We can unschedule a little time each day to just play with our kids. Maybe we can teach our kids to throw a ball in the yard rather than sign them up for T-ball. Our kids love being with us, especially when we are willing to get outside and have a little adventure together. Perhaps we can get some of our own exercise by riding around the neighbourhood with our kids, by playing frisbee in the park together or working together as neighbours to open the gym in the winter for games like dodge ball and pick-up basket-ball. It takes courage and confidence to rebel against the tide of non-stop programming of our children's time.

What if we do miss a window of opportunity for our child's special talents—what if they join the soccer league two years later than the other kids? Let's not forget that kids can still be active; they can still learn about music and reading and throwing a ball with their parents. We are so certain that other people are the experts in these areas, but perhaps we are better qualified than anybody to play with our own kids.

Sometimes in the middle of the day I want to take my five-year-old and meet a friend for coffee with her daughter—but her daughter has dance lessons or choir practice, or my friend is simply too busy to get out of the house for a couple of hours. Her schedule combined with my own means we actually need our electonic organizers just to plan a coffee date!

Parenting today can be an isolating experience. When we suddenly have to get milk or medicine, or to take our son to the doctor, chances are we bundle up the whole family and take them with us. If we are going crazy listening to the strange and wonderful language of two-year-olds all day, we likely have to wait until our partner or a friend comes home from work to be able to connect with an adult. My neighbours probably would take my kids if I asked for help, but I rarely do. On the odd occasion that I have thought to ask for help, nobody is home. People aren't in their houses today as much as they are in their cars, driving to lessons, home from work, to the next child-centred event.

There is a better way. We and our children don't have to continue at this unbearable pace. Our kids need us to take some of the pressure off their schedules and off ourselves. We don't have to be doing everything right to be great parents; we just need to be with our kids, loving them, spending time with them, finding things we can do together as families and as communities.

We love our kids and we deserve this time with them. We are not simply chauffeurs and family administrators: we are their best friends and role models.

When I lead capture-the-flag once a week in our neighbourhood park, I am taking time to be with other people's kids as well as my own. My son loves that I lead this game, just as he loves when I volunteer at school. I am showing him that I am a willing participant in his world, and the fact that I am having fun delights him. It is important that I am present and enjoying myself rather than showing up just because I should—kids can tell the difference. Last summer, I spent a day at the waterslides with my children. William and I went up the big slides together over and over again. I found the slides thrilling, and screamed and laughed my way down each time. He would go first and then wait at the bottom to watch me plunge into the water. By the time I surfaced, we would both be laughing with glee, and each time we headed up the hill again he would grab my hand and, in an excited voice, plan our next trip down. I was so thankful that I had made the decision to play rather than to sit in the shade and read my book. In the midst of our busy lives, it is important not to forget that we volunteer at their schools, play with them after dinner and show up for important moments in their lives not because it is our obligation, but because we *want* to—because we delight in watching their triumphs and supporting them through challenges. We love our kids and we deserve this time with them. We are not simply chauffeurs and family administrators: we are their best friends and role models.

Dave Steen, a Commonwealth gold medal–winning shot putter, is a passionate advocate for healthy families:

> Two powerful myths afoot in modern culture are that we can have it all and we can get it with little effort. Well, let's get real. We can't have everything, so we have to make wise choices. The first is our families—loving and nurturing our kids. Part of that is making sure

they're physically active and well nourished—
every day. There are no shortcuts in this. It
takes time and smart planning and follow-
through. These good habits must last a lifetime, both theirs and yours.

Our children are sponges. They pick up our attitudes toward our bodies and our attitudes and rou-
tines regarding health and physical activity. I've always
told my children that breakfast is an important start
to the day, but a year ago Kate asked me, "Mommy,
why don't *you* eat breakfast?" Never a morning eater,
I've been choking down scrambled eggs and fruit with
them every morning since. I can't expect them to
believe that breakfast is important if I don't eat it
myself. My girlfriend's little girl walks to school
swinging her arms and moving her legs at full speed.
One day, when I asked her what she was doing, she
said, "I'm power-walking," which is exactly what her
mom does every day. What we do has a far more powerful impact than what we say, and what we do
together *as a family* has a profound impact on our children's beliefs, attitudes and behaviour. Sometimes we
forget that our children are learning everything for
the first time and that we as parents are their primary
teachers. My daughter told me, "I'm going to row,
Mommy," not because she had seen pictures of me

rowing at the Olympics, but because she spent time at the lake watching her mom's masters rowing team. We leave lasting impressions on them with everything we do. The examples we set of healthy eating and exercising—and, most importantly, what we do together as a family—are the real opportunities we have to excite and inspire our children to live well.

If children are going to have a lifelong love of physical movement and a healthy relationship with their bodies, then this relationship needs to unfold in the family setting. How we take care of ourselves, what we do together as a family and what we eat are all keenly observed by our kids. It seems that more and more we look to external influences—schools and social infrastructure, community centres and soccer pitches—to provide our children with what they ought to be getting at home. Everything that happens out in our communities should be considered as support to what we do at home, not a replacement for family activity and our being role models. Shelley Landsberg, a community health nurse working on St. Mary's Reserve in New Brunswick, says,

> I used to think that [family and individual health] was as simple as providing the environment to install these healthy programs, and

then people would just participate in them. I'm not convinced of that anymore. I think a lot of what's going on in any community has more to do with bigger, more abstract things than just having the activity program in the community or having the healthy snack initiative because when the child leaves school, they go back into their communities, into their home and into their family life, and if those areas are not making behavioural or lifestyle changes, then what is learned at school gets lost or forgotten or consciously abandoned. Do you eat in front of the TV or do you sit down as a family? Does somebody cook healthy meals in the family or do you eat takeout food? Does the family go for walks together; is exercise part of the family life?

When parents are active with their kids, kids love being active. Watch toddlers for a few hours and you will observe that they are always exploring and testing their physical limits. They want to move, and we usually get the most resistance when we try to interrupt that movement. Any of us who have experienced "board-boy phenomenon" while struggling to get a two-year-old into his car seat can relate to how forcefully a two-year-old will resist being stuck. Our role as parents is to support and encourage our children's natural desire to move.

When it comes to doing activities together as a family, parents need to find things that their kids love to do and do those things with them. While I love power-walking, that is not something a child particularly wants to do for fun. Children like things that are more short-burst anaerobic activity (like tag or hide and seek) because it suits their attention spans and imaginations. Dr. Gabriela Tymowski, the director of LEAP!, shared the following:

> We have some parents who tell us, "We went out on a thirty-kilometre bike ride, but she always gets so tired and can't keep up." Well, the response there is that the parents need to slow down and do some things with their child that are just with and for their child. These things appear to be quite obvious or common-sensical, but the families just don't seem to understand it and I don't know if it's because they have forgotten what it's like to be a child. Parents are running around trying to make the best lives possible for their children, but they're missing the big picture. What their kids really want is for somebody to go for a bike ride with them at their speed rather than being dropped

off somewhere or left behind. We have one little boy in the [pediatric obesity] program whose parents drop him off at the soccer field and they don't understand why he's over-weight. They say, "He plays soccer all the time," but it turns out he's the goalie so he just stands there on his own. He's not with the team and they're not there to even notice that. They just drop him off and think they've done their duty.

When speaking with Dr. Tymowski, I learned that there is a fairly constant and reliable set of behaviours in families with overweight or obese children: they don't eat meals together, and they often have TVs in every room in the house. "Three-quarters of the kids in our program eat dinner at home, alone, in their bedrooms while watching TV," she explained. "It's really scary. There are families for whom physical activity is not part of their routine and families who tend to reward behaviour with food. Families who tend to be super-busy and eat a lot of packaged food or fast food; families who have no real identifiable interests, who don't do things as a family. TV is a huge one, and not eating family meals is common across the board."

Most parents I have spoken to feel confused about how much to feed their kids, what to feed them and what is strictly off limits. We live in a world filled with emotionally charged information about avoiding trans fats, eating limited carbohydrates, drinking soy milk, choosing non-genetically altered foods. Information about what we should eat assaults us from every corner. We have health food stores telling us that we need to eat organic, that sugar is "white death," that the meat we buy is full of growth hormones and antibiotics. That doesn't sound good. And the dialogue expands to encompass how to cook food to maintain its nutrients, how much fish oil you need in your diet, the suggestion that we shun all animal fats.

There are valid points to all of the above, but for a busy parent, it's just too much information. In addition, this information is often presented by non-neutral sources such as food companies, dairy boards and marketers of low-fat products. If you are like me, sometimes you just don't know what you should eat and you are even more confused about what you should feed your kids.

My philosophy on food is—keep it simple. In the world of nutrition this is remarkably difficult to do. Yet it's important to make the effort, and there are a few ideas that have helped me enormously in feeding my kids. Canada's Food Guide is an excellent resource that reminds me about the variety of foods kids need to be healthy. At each meal, I provide a vegetable, a grain and a meat or alternative. It doesn't take a lot of fancy planning to do this, but how we shop is essential to our success. If it's not in the fridge, we can't eat it. If I buy potato chips, I will eat them. If I have healthy vegetables in

Do as much of your shopping as you can in the outside aisles of the grocery store.

my crisper, that's what I'll eat. We simply need to remind ourselves that kids need vegetables, good-quality grains, and proteins. As for drinks, juice, Gatorade-type drinks and pop have a lot of sugar and calories, so we drink juice only once a day. For three years, my son whined, "I hate water." Personally, I can't grasp how you can hate something that is tasteless, colourless and odourless, but that's the mystery of kids. Now he drinks water without complaint because no alternatives are offered (except "water with ice").

I also avoid foods with a lot of ingredients in them. Packaged foods, pre-made dinners and frozen pizzas are not a big part of my family's diet. These foods tend to have a lot of artificial ingredients and are laden with salt and sugar. Not only that, but labels can often be misleading. For instance, it is not yet required to state that foods contain trans fats, and bakery and deli items often do not have lists of ingredients. Sometimes, what seems to be an innocent—even healthy—snack is really pretty bad for us. There are many parents who have been led to believe that those little fish-shaped crackers are a healthy snack for their kids, but they need to be moved into the once-in-a-while category.

As an athlete, I learned a fair amount about nutrition, but the most useful piece of advice I ever got was to try to do as much of your shopping as you can in the outside aisles of the grocery store. At my grocery store, the fruits and vegetables are along one side; the back aisle of the store has dairy products, eggs, and the fish market; and the other outside aisle has the meat section, followed by the bread section. I get most of my groceries in the outside aisles and then I do a quick jaunt to the inside aisles for extras like canned tomatoes, rice, pasta, jam and maybe a bag of cookies. I also avoid economy- or family-sized packages because they seem to encourage me to buy foods I would not normally purchase. I made this decision after returning from Wal-Mart one day with what looked to be a year's supply of nacho chips. Recently, I have even distilled the routine of shopping to going once every six weeks to a butcher who carries free-range and non-steroid-laden meat, once every two weeks to my regular grocery store for supplies and once every few days to the fruit and vegetable store down the street.

It all sounds so easy, doesn't it? *If* we can ignore the cries for "Cheezies, Cheezies" from our two-year-old as we walk down the grocery aisle ... The cry is persistent and, well, rather loud, so we reach for the Cheezies and open the bag. Ah, peace again! This works pretty well: one little treat to make up for half an hour of being lugged around a grocery store—it even seems fair. As kids get older, they have opinions on everything: what cereal they want, what juices their friends drink, that their lunches are so boring, that they "don't want to eat healthy food ANY MORE!" This tests our mettle, and we are determined to hold out—only healthy food in my house, not a single trans fat in their bodies—and then we realize: we are weak, they are strong. We need to compromise.

We are in a junk-food war, where every birthday party, every school fundraising event, every special occasion is a battleground full of unhealthy food.

That is what real life looks like. So, except for products that have so many artificial ingredients or so much caffeine in them that I think of them as poison, I allow my kids to eat everything—everything, that is, once in a while. I ask them to make a list of once-in-a-while foods they like to have. Each shopping trip I buy them one of these items. My kids' lists have included processed cheese strings, Minigos, Froot Loops, Cheezies, ice cream and cookies. But I also get them to make a list of healthy foods they would like me to buy. This week my son's list included French vanilla yogourt, raspberries and fresh pasta. I usually do the main grocery shopping at night, when my kids are sleeping. This allows me to take their lists and get a few of their once-in-a-while foods without being constantly barraged with their pleas for this candy or that juice. It's well worth paying a babysitter for an hour! I allow them to go to the fruit and vegetable store with me every couple of days because, frankly, I can live with pretty much every choice they make there.

Good food can be expensive, and I think it is time that governments encouraged both healthy eating and good community planning so that, for instance, convenience stores aren't the only shopping option within walking distance of a disadvantaged neighbourhood. Every child, regardless of his or her economic situation, deserves access to healthy food.

And so there it is. I am doing the best I can in a far-from-perfect world. The rest of the battle of keeping good food in our children's bodies requires us to attain warrior status. We are in a junk-food war, where every birthday party, every school fundraising event, every special occasion is a battleground full of unhealthy food. The arrows consist of pop, candy and pizza, and little rolls with sausages in them. I lift my shield to repel these arrows, but the onslaught is so relentless it begins to wear me down.

I don't even know why parties and fairs and fundraisers are called "special events" anymore. They happen every weekend, and every week in school. Teachers can't always make special rules covering how our kids eat at such events or in the classroom because the events themselves often dictate what's being consumed. Pizza day, hot dog day and cupcake sales are regular occurences in many schools. I have a few rules that I am sure have given me the status of "food police" in some other parents' eyes. No pop. Full of sugar, loaded with caffeine, tons of calories—just no. Eat before we go to the party. This we often do, and it curbs the amount of junk that is consumed at birthday celebrations. Other than that, I don't know what to do that won't label my kids and me as just plain fanatical. (Of course, I'm probably already labelled, so maybe I shouldn't worry about it.) But as I mentioned, warrior status is what's needed if we really want to affect how our kids eat. In Port Williams elementary school in Nova Scotia, one parent, Jane Holmes, worked with teachers to create a healthy food policy and managed to get pop and fast food out of her children's school. She has inspired me to work with others to ensure that my children's school doesn't raise money by selling food that is bad for our kids' health.

But I cling to the fact that if my kids move enough, a little bit of sugary, fatty food is not going to kill them. The best approach to making sure our kids reach a healthy weight and get adequate nutrition is to keep them moving. When they are moving, they don't have a chance to overeat; and when they are moving, they are pretty hungry by the time they are called for dinner. Hungry kids are more likely to eat the salad you put in front of them than are kids who have spent the two hours before dinner sitting at the computer.

Dr. Tymowski says, "Maintaining a healthy weight is a pretty straightforward equation: energy in must equal energy out, but it seems that—even just anec-dotally—that isn't as common a knowledge as I thought!" Her LEAP! program is focused on using education to help children and their families make healthy decisions about eating and physical activity. According to Dr. Tymowski, combatting obesity in a child requires the commitment of the whole family: "For parents, we tell them that in order to see change, the whole family has to be involved. It is unrealistic to come to a clinic once a month and expect the child to have lost weight. Parents play an integral role in being role models, supporting their kids and going out and doing things with them instead of telling them to go out and do things."

Obesity is also not just an eating issue; it is a negative energy equation, and in children the healthiest approach is to focus on the activity levels and, rather than limit food, make healthier choices on the food being eaten. Our children's being overweight harms them in profound and lasting ways. When asked about the ethical issues of childhood obesity, Dr. Tymowski becomes even more passionate:

> Children have a right to an open future, that they should arrive on the cusp of adulthood ready to take anything on. Obesity forecloses their futures in many ways. For one, it means they didn't have a normal childhood. It also means they are dealing with depression, low self-esteem and lack of confidence. It means they will likely have *never* participated in sport or an organized physical activity program; they probably don't have many outside interests. I argue that children who are obese are being harmed, and this is not a very politically correct thing to say, but parents are the first line with regards to the issue of responsibility. They are the ones charged with the responsibility of making sure their children are happy and healthy.

—

Clearly, childhood obesity and being overweight are no longer issues we can allow ourselves to ignore.

Both Dr. Andrew Pipe and Dr. Tymowski believe that our children's weight problems have been overlooked because there are so many overweight kids that if our kids are a little heavy, it just seems normal. Dr. Tymowski contends that the number of overweight kids is quite a bit higher than the published statistics show, because in surveys people self-report their weight, and always underestimate. Dr. Mark Tremblay pointed out this gap between perception and reality—an Angus Reid report says about 12% of parents believe their kids to be overweight, but when the children were actually measured, 27% were overweight.

I asked Dr. Tymowski to help me understand what the obese children who come to her clinic are feeling. She talked to me about their low self-esteem, their low energy levels and the depression she sees directly related to their obesity. She also cited a study that came out a few years ago that showed obese children feel worse psychologically than kids who have cancer. They feel the prognosis for their lives is more miserable than it would be if they had *cancer*. Obesity affects kids in the home, at school, in their friendships. No child deserves to feel this hopeless about life.

Is it right or acceptable for children as young as

five years old to be talking about going on diets? Should the primary goal of a child that young be to lose weight? As parents and as a society, can we live with the knowledge that thousands of our children, the lights of our future, are struggling with depression, anxiety and weak bodies?

It is true that we are being aggressively marketed to by the makers of convenience foods, that it is more difficult than ever for kids to be active at school, that all of us parents are increasingly stretched and stressed. However, the truth remains that what happens in our families is the most important factor in the health of our children. As Dr. Tymowski explains, "It is a pretty unpopular thing to say, but I see the solution to the epidemic of obesity starting in the home. Only you can buy the groceries for your kids; only you can help your kids understand how to make better decisions."

I was at the Ministry of Health in Ottawa last fall and was appalled—utterly appalled—to see that the off-hours cafeteria food was 98% absolute junk. I'm talking Wagon Wheels, chocolate bars, Twinkies. I didn't know they still made Twinkies! If this junk is at the Ministry of Health, it really *is* everywhere. We have to find the time to learn about what is healthy, and we have to stay strongly committed to eating well inside and outside the home. I am not saying it is easy; it absolutely isn't. But what our kids eat is a critical part of keeping them healthy, and it is *our* job to ensure that they do.

Being a parent today is an exercise in vigilance. I remember installing my first infant car seat. There was a large manual that talked about locking clips and rear-facing placement, asked for the weight of the child, instructed me to keep the handle down while driving. It just seemed so complicated. There are studies

> As parents, it's useful to know why our kids have to be active, but all our kids need to know is that they are having fun.

and instructions and experts and debates and graphs and statistics for everything we do, and we long for someone to distill the information so that we can more easily figure out the best course of action.

Well, the experts are telling us that our children need sixty cumulative minutes of physical activity a day for optimal development. (I have read that it's ninety minutes, but I wonder if governments and health promotion agencies have lowered it to sixty to make it more attainable.) This means sixty minutes of movement that gets the heart pumping and the bones loaded. If we translate this into an hour on the Stairmaster or running, it sounds unachievable. But in kids' terms, this means time spent riding a bike, twenty minutes walking to school or in the evening with us, an hour outside playing hoops or soccer or inline skating. As parents, it's useful to know why our kids have to be active, but all our kids need to know is that they are having fun.

Adopting the approach of getting serious about play sets a totally different tone than getting serious about fitness. One sounds like work, the other like a whole lot of fun. I don't want to talk to my kids about getting fit; I just want to create opportunities for them to move. As Dr. Tymowski says, maintaining a healthy weight can be seen as an equation between energy in and energy out. With children, energy out is the part that is the most fun for us to focus on. I think it is good to give kids information about what adequate activity is doing for their bodies, but it is very important that kids don't feel as if they are exercising just to be healthy. This can too easily become yet another thing that they have to do. Moving is fun, and it is our challenge as parents and educators to help kids find ways of moving that are engaging and joyful.

I passionately believe that fun must be the centre of physical activity for our kids. And since we're talking about fun, let's not forget adults. Grown-ups can be motivated by long-term goals such as taking off weight or lowering the chance of heart disease, but my observation is that an exercise program that is fun is an exercise program that works and that people stick

with. Adults who find enjoyable ways of keeping fit—
dancing and walking and playing hockey with the
gang—hardly recognize they are exercising and are
far more likely to stick with it than those who force
themselves to go to the gym three times a week to get
into shape.

The number one thing that activity brings me today
is joy. Hands down, no question—I don't even have to
think about it. When I climb a mountain, when I
walk in the rain, when I finish those last poses in yoga,
I experience joy. For two decades, I trained my body
to be an efficient rowing machine. Training could be
an incredible high, and I would often be filled with
adrenaline, purpose and feelings of accomplishment. I
would also experience the physiological high of
endorphins coursing through my system, the vibrancy
of a strong body, the endurance of well-trained muscles. Even though a lot of what I did was hard, I loved
it. I loved the feeling of the boat moving through
water, and I had so much fun being part of a team.
But just as often, I pushed through fatigue and pain,
reminding myself that the physical discomfort was
temporary and would bring rewards.

Today I don't have the goal of winning an
Olympic medal, so I am less willing to push myself
into oxygen deprivation and extreme muscle fatigue. I

no longer exercise at the intensity that creates burning in my lungs and cramping in my legs. I am still willing to push through some fatigue and muscle soreness, I am still willing to get past my first position in yoga into a deeper pose, but mostly the exercise itself has to be enjoyable. I have to enjoy most parts of power-walking around the lake, most parts of lifting myself into a handstand, or I simply won't do it. Playing hockey with the guys once a week is more likely to last a decade than is meeting up with the Stairmaster every Wednesday. Similarly, the reason I love walking is that I can walk with a close friend and get caught up on our lives—we have such a good time that we forget about our ten-kilometre commitment until it's over. When I can walk alone, I experience a meditative state. We need to find activities that we enjoy. If it isn't fun, it is too much like hard work.

Many parents struggle to find a window of time for their own exercise. But sometimes integrating family time and exercise time really works. I will power-walk beside my five-year-old as she rides. When I am watching William at soccer practice, I will run around the field with Kate, once in a while dropping to the ground to do push-ups. The emergence of fitness boot camps here in Victoria has made this a little more socially acceptable; I have even been asked by one mom if I would consider running a camp while the children play. My friend Laurie Anne is already doing this. While her kids play soccer, she pulls all the parents together into an outdoor workout group and they run and do push-ups and dips. This is certainly conveying a powerful message to the kids: parents are active too.

I believe we have to look at ourselves and ask what barriers we are creating that keep our children from enjoying family play. Parents tell me that a shortage of hours in the day is the biggest obstacle to family time.

Some of my best weekends with my kids are "No Agenda Weekends," when we don't have to be anywhere or do anything.

In addition to a long day at school, many children have increased homework due to changes in the curriculum. As well, many of us feel pressure to give our kids a head start in learning. With the grade-point averages needed for university entrance getting higher, our kids' doing well academically has become progressively more important. It is common to have "tween" children working with a tutor or taking an extra academic subject such as French after school. All of this adds up to less time for movement, both in the schools and out.

I sometimes feel overwhelmed by all the things I am supposed to do to give my kids a "head start." As they get older, I realize how little family time there really is: between school, homework and activities, kids can easily be apart from their family for almost the entire day. Time spent driving them to lessons is great, but nothing compares to having my daughter delight in the chestnut she finds as we walk around the block together. I want this time, and I am willing to go against the norm in order to get it. We take the dog for a walk after supper because it is a fabulous opportunity to

Building unstructured time back into our family life sometimes seems counter-intuitive: we need to be less active to be more active.

talk. While my kids are young, I refuse to give up every weekend to hockey practice, piano recitals and birthday parties. I want time to take my kids swimming or to do yardwork while they play in the driveway.

Some of my best weekends with my kids are "No Agenda Weekends," when we don't have to be anywhere or do anything. Last weekend I asked both my kids what would make a great day for them. Kate asked to bake cookies and set up a roadside stand to sell them. William wanted me to kick the ball outside with him for at least an hour. They both asked to meet a friend for a play date. We walked through the neighbourhood on our way to breakfast. After breakfast we came back home and read books. I did yoga while the kids turned my kitchen into a lunar landing pad. The day felt slow and luxurious, although we moved through many different activities (baking, walking, lunar landing, cleaning, breakfast, bike riding). I want more days like these, days where I resist the temptation to drive somewhere or to turn on the television for the kids.

In my family, we have made a conscious effort not to get the kids involved in more than one structured activity a week. We try to free up time in the morning for homework so that in the evening we can focus on family and community play. This sounds very organized, but what it really means is taking the dog for a walk, finding a neighbourhood friend to play in the park with or, on cold and wet days, transforming the garage into a hockey rink. I remember as a child being allowed to play floor hockey in our small basement. It was a huge amount of fun and there seemed to be ample room. As an adult, I look back and think my parents were pretty relaxed, letting us smash balls around like that, and I thank them for being that way. We also had pogo sticks, which we used in the basement when it was minus twenty outside.

Building unstructured time back into our family life sometimes seems counterintuitive: we need to be less active to be more active. I am certainly not suggesting that we stop all organized sports and activities, but I *am* advocating that we pull back in order to create the time for families to be active together. With more time spent in our own neighbourhoods, we shift the focus of our families and communities. If we come together and agree that Wednesday is family and community playtime, the chances of our children having others to play with are far greater. The time we spend riding our bikes or playing basketball with other neighbourhood kids is some of the best quality time my kids and I spend together.

When my siblings and I were growing up, there was a sort of collective eye on all of us kids. We played outside on the street, and no one in particular—yet everyone—was watching us. Today, while we prepare dinner, our kids are inside with us (too often watching television). This is something we can change, and we can begin by meeting our neighbours and discovering ways our kids can play together.

Speaking of television, screen time—spent with video games, television programs and computer games and in chat rooms—is a formidable opponent to our children's well-being. No matter how good the program or game, and even if there is a strong educational component, it is still on a screen. Sedentary, unrealistic and completely absorbing, these screens know how to capture our kids.

I am a single parent of two kids, and like every

other parent I know, I have put my kids in front of the television or allowed them to play a computer game because I need to make dinner. And there have been Friday afternoons when I've happily napped while they played Need for Speed or Zoo Tycoon. These activities are all fun, but I'd hesitate to consider them play. Boys seem to be particularly drawn to video games that have them driving at high speeds around corners, shooting villains and creating imaginary cities. I admit to enjoying these games myself: my son and I have a great time racing each other or creating cities. There are also a lot of really well-written TV shows for kids. Yes, I can rationalize that the game they are playing or the show they are watching is educational, but the truth is I just need some time. The problem is that "some time" can so easily become a lot of time— an hour, maybe even two. With only a few hours an evening to spend as a family, we have to be careful not to let those screens steal our time.

Screens may be entertaining, but they are not presenting a realistic paradigm. They are about instant feedback, instant gratification and high-speed information. But the world doesn't work that way. It takes effort to get results; it takes time to understand a problem. I worry about all the friends that kids are making on MSN, people they often know nothing about—if they picked up the phone to talk to them, or if they met them in person, they might have a totally different impression of them. This is not to say I believe that everything on computer screens is bad, or that connecting through the Internet is never a good option. I support a program called Ability Online that connects housebound kids with chronic illness and disabilities with one another. I have witnessed how the computer can be an important link from one child with a debilitating condition to another—it is truly inspiring to see how electronic connections can dissipate feelings of isolation.

We can work with our children to create realistic and agreed upon limits regarding screen time, but we can't expect them to limit themselves.

As a parent, I have found that establishing a set amount of cumulative screen time is an effective compromise. My kids know they are allowed a total of two hours of screen time during the week and can use those two hours pretty much as they wish. This might mean that one day they watch an hour of television and the next day they spend half an hour on the computer. On the weekend they are allowed an hour a day. But this weekend we were so busy doing other things we didn't have time to watch television, and neither of the kids has even mentioned it.

I have heard parents say, "I just can't get my son away from Xbox." I say, turn it off. If it can't be turned off, it leaves the house. In my family, it is not all about what the children want—sometimes what they want is simply not good for them. We can work with our children to create realistic and agreed-upon limits regarding screen time, but we can't expect them to limit themselves. *We* are the adults, and it's up to us to create and enforce rules. My girlfriend Kim said that fights over what games to play on Xbox caused a near riot in her household. After several warnings to her two boys, she did a brave and radical thing. She yelled, "Enough!"—in a voice every parent would recognize—then unplugged the Xbox and dragged it to the car. Her boys looked at her blankly, not really comprehending what their mother was doing. She sold the Xbox that very same day and donated the money to tsunami relief. The aftermath of her actions included an entire month of sulking from her oldest son. A year later, she believes her family life has changed for the better. "We play games together, we have so much more family time, and when the boys say they are bored, a few minutes later they have found something to do," she tells me. In some families, selling the Xbox wouldn't be a realistic option—I realize that. But limits *can* be created and respected.

We can't expect an eight-year-old to understand

the long-term consequences of watching television three hours a night; it would be difficult to explain to him that he is building a habit, not being active, and chiselling away at family time. We can't expect our kids to understand this, the same way we can't expect them to make healthy food choices given the opportunity to eat Cheezies and french fries for dinner each day. Perhaps eventually they will understand why we have imposed limits, but for now we lead the way.

In his book *Finding Flow*, Mihaly Csikszentmihalyi studies peak experiences, or "flow." He contends that people experience good feelings most often when they are intrinsically motivated to do something, when they have a goal for doing it and when the thing they are doing requires an initial investment of energy. His psychological study of how people spend their time reveals that kids and adults do not experience flow when they are watching television or playing video games. Without exception, they experience flow during an activity that requires an initial investment of energy—going for a run, climbing a hill, playing the guitar. In other words, he's saying what most adults know: that we have to work a little to experience the truly remarkable in life—great moments don't come unless we set the conditions for them to come. Our kids simply can't understand this, but they *can* feel the joy of kicking a soccer ball. While we were playing a quick game of soccer, parents against kids, one of the little boys on William's team said to me, "This is way more fun than playing Xbox." I'll tell you, in this world, that is the kind of encouragement I need to hear. It is the little bit of real-life evidence that gives me hope and shows me that we are on the right track when we create opportunities for our kids to be active and engaged in life.

Yesterday, I told the kids we were spending the afternoon hiking. My son moaned, "I don't want to go hiking, it's so boooring." I wanted to get fresh air, so I was motivated to get us on that hike. So I said to him, "Okay, William, what if we asked some friends to come along with us?" Suddenly it was "Yippee, we are going hiking!" I called a girlfriend, and we piled in two of her children, my two and two of the neighbour's kids and drove to a great trail a few kilometres away. Once at the trail, all six of the kids raced ahead, screaming and shouting when they saw that there was ice on the inlet, making a lot of noise and having a lot of fun. We walked, talked and ran for two and a half hours, kids ranging from three to eight years old running circles around us. It was worth it to think my way past William's initial resistance.

As I mentioned earlier, kids don't always like the same activities their parents do. We need to put aside our own athletic agendas when trying to be active with our kids. Some of this has been hard for me: I'd love to cycle twenty kilometres with my kids, but I usually settle for cycling to the park and then spending an hour playing there. It is also important to pay attention to our children's capabilities. When I take children hiking, I want every one of them to have a positive experience. This may mean that we go half the distance I originally planned because little Ashley is having trouble keeping up. It often means we sing songs, tell stories and look for treasures along the way.

We always need to balance our own expectations of what a child can do with what the child actually is capable of doing. The line between encouraging our children to try something new and pushing them too hard is a pretty fine one. If children have been inactive, physical activity will be harder for them, and, unlike adults, they can't really grasp that their muscles and lungs may hurt for a while to get into condition. Children live so much in the present that the idea of working hard for benefits later can be a tough sell, which is why it is far better to focus on activities that are fun.

So will my kids miss their Olympic opportunity if they are not seriously involved in sports for the first decade of their life? No. I did a casual poll of my rowing team and discovered that out of twenty-two athletes, only four had competed seriously in sports before the age of ten. Most of them had done school sports, but many hadn't even been "athletic" until their high school years. Canadian Olympic cyclist Lori-Ann Munzer didn't start cycling until she was twenty-two, and won a gold medal at the age of thirty-eight. She says, "Your age is only a number on your driver's licence."

When I work with my children to find activities that capture their imagination and challenge them, I am teaching them one of the most important life skills: how to be fully engaged. They are figuring out how to keep themselves busy when they feel bored; they are learning that effort translates into increased competence, and that increased competence leads to increased enjoyment. I want my kids to have dreams, and to possess the discipline needed to fulfill those dreams. If they can look at life and see its adventure and challenge and magic, they will be well on their way. These are the things that I believe play and sport can teach kids. We need to help our children develop these abilities so that they can move into adulthood knowing how to help themselves feel good and knowing what maximizes their chances of living an outstanding life.

Let's not make physical activity too complicated. Let's rejoice in the fact that our kids want to move, and encourage them to jump a little more, wrestle a little more, run outside roaring.

Fun Things You Can Do with Your Family

Kick a soccer ball

Throw a football

Play catch with a baseball

Blow bubbles and try to pop them before they land

Invite neighbourhood kids to play in your yard

Ride bikes together

Walk the dog together

Go out at night and search for stars or constellations

Find those neighbourhood kids and offer to supervise a game
of capture-the-flag

Skip rope (some have built-in counters that kids love)

Climb a tree

Meet neighbours in a local park

Offer to supervise a space once a week where kids can gather
and play

In bad weather, clear some space in the house and play red
light, green light

Wrestle together

Go to family swim time at the local pool

Go to the community centre or the local school

Start a neighbourhood basketball night

Do an indoor scavenger hunt

Create a scavenger hunt in your neighbourhood

Create a scavenger hunt in your apartment building

Get out the pillows and do gymnastics

Turn on the music and have an evening dance club

Pull the car out of the garage and play garage hockey

Run up the stairs in your apartment building and keep track of
    who has done the most flights

Sidestep in the hallways of your apartment building

Keep balls, skipping ropes and frisbees in your car

Invest in pedometers and track your family's increase in steps

Race your kids to the car

Play Twister

Play tag

Play kick-the-can

Have a hula-hoop contest

Do somersaults in the living room

Walk the curb

Do yoga

Jump for joy

Fly a kite

Walk to the video store

Walk to school

Park a few blocks from your destination and walk the rest of
    the way

Create an obstacle course for bikes

Use a stopwatch to time your kids running around the house

Choreograph an aerobics class for kids

Play keep-away

Keep a balloon in the air

"The sport we live is, or ought to be, an authentic expression of the values we hold most dear."

RIC YOUNG

THE SPORT WE WANT

Tiger Woods's dad had him practising his short game at the age of four. In 1997, Woods became the youngest man ever to wear golf's coveted green jacket, winning the Masters at twenty-one. The greatest gymnast of all time, Nadia Comaneci, was taken to a specialized training school at the tender age of six and went on to win five Olympic medals, including three golds, at the Montreal Olympics. When Wayne Gretzky was six, his dad built him a rink in the back-yard. By the age of ten, when he scored an unprece-dented 378 goals in his last year of peewee, Gretzky was recognized as a hockey prodigy.

As parents, we want to give our children every chance of succeeding. Whether we admit it or not, some of us dream of our kids playing in the NHL or bringing home a medal for Canada. Most of all, we don't want to limit our kids. That window of opportunity in music or sports or academics that will make the difference between our kids being good or great is a window we are afraid of missing. We might not want to push them into sports or music, but we certainly don't want to discover when they are ten that they have a talent and might have been extraordinary had we developed it earlier. I want what everybody else wants: for my children to be fully equipped to realize their potential in whatever they have a passion for.

But I think we might be getting a little neurotic. Parents regularly ask me for advice on what they should be doing to produce great athletes—"I think my daughter is really talented. What's the best rowing club for her?" or "How many hours a week should my eight-year-old daughter be practising diving?" They tell me about a select diving program their child is in that has them practising three days a week, or a gold-level soccer team that they would like their son to try out for.

Perhaps we are getting the idea that children have to start organized high-level sport early to maximize their potential, that all great athletes start their sports in the early years. This might be true for a sport like gymnastics, where athletes peak at eighteen, but it is certainly not true for the majority of sports. My informal survey of dozens of Olympic athletes gleaned responses like that of kayaker Adam van Koeverdan, who told me he did everything, but nothing in particular, until age thirteen, when his mom signed him up for the kayak club to keep him out of trouble. Gymnast Kyle Shewfelt, who did begin training at age six, also remembers getting much of his fitness and dexterity on the backyard trampoline. Basketball great Steve Nash's parents said Steve grew up playing every sport. He played on soccer and basketball teams, but also played street hockey, capture-the-flag and any other conceivable game with the neighbourhood kids. His sister, Joann, told me that whenever they felt bored, they had only to look out the window to find someone to play with. My experience competing in four Olympic games and befriending hundreds of top athletes along the way is that the common thread through their athletic development is an active childhood of physical play and sports.

When parents approach me for advice on raising champions, a huge part of me just wants to say, "Relax. Relax and just let your kids play!" We need to remember to enjoy our kids, and stop worrying that we are doing the wrong things.

In some ways, we *are* doing the wrong things—but not in the ways we thought. I see four-years-olds trying to follow the rules of a soccer game; it is painful for the coach trying to teach them, as well as frustrating for the kids, who simply are not cognitively ready to follow complex instructions. What they should be doing is kicking and running and *playing*.

> Children six and under aren't really cognitively ready to play sports with complex rules and strategies.

It is very easy for a young child to assume she doesn't like soccer if she is asked to follow rules that are too complicated or is upset by a parent yelling, "Defence! Defence!" on the sidelines of a league game. Research shows that kids drop out of sport when they feel stress, when there is a mismatching of ability to challenge or when they perceive criticism. My son told me how he felt about my vocal "encouragement" quite early on. While cycling up a steep hill together, I shouted, "Pump your legs, pump your legs!" He burst into tears, asking, "Why are you yelling at me?" It is so important at this age that we don't project our adult perceptions of sport onto our children. Let them play, learn some new skills and make friends.

There is substantial research that shows that children six and under aren't really cognitively ready to play sports with complex rules and strategies. They literally are built for *play* at this age, needing to experience a large range of activities and unable to concentrate on any one of them for too long. Any of us who have coached five-year-olds playing soccer, where kids run like a swarm of bees behind the ball, know that rules and strategy are not a productive focus for this age group. The kids want to play, and although they are developmentally and physically highly receptive to learning new skills, this has to be done in a fun context, with lots of repetition.

Between the ages of six and nine, structured and unstructured activities should be fun and children should be developing agility, balance, coordination and speed: the ABCS of physical literacy. The ABCS are developed through running, jumping, throwing, kicking, catching and twisting. Playing a variety of sports and enjoying highly physical outdoor play will help your child reach optimal physical development.

Just as we have learned enormous amounts over the past decade about how children's brains develop, so we now know a lot more about how their bodies develop in various stages. Many of the athletic associations in this country are now using sound research about athletic development to tailor their programs to these windows of learning and physical development that children experience. But as parents, we must balance what science tells us with what seems sensible and appropriate for our own children and families.

It is my hope that the information on physical, emotional and social development will help coaches and PE teachers tailor their games and sport programs too, to better suit children's windows of development as well as their physical, emotional and social needs. My fear is that we will take the information so literally that we will become obsessed with making the most of each window of development and forget that kids do most of what this science is teaching us when they are active in the schoolyard and in the neighbourhood.

Our kids are great, every one of them, gifted with their own unique talents and abilities—but those talents and abilities evolve over time.

I'll say it again: there is nobody more qualified than you to play with your kids; coaches and teachers will help them develop their skills, but the time you take as a family to throw a ball, swim together and learn to bowl will give your kids the high-quality family time they long for and give them a great start in many varied activities.

—

I believe our obsession with ensuring our kids don't miss out on their chance at greatness has contributed to an unbearable amount of stress on our kids and our families. We are all in this pressure cooker of high expectations, so driven to give our kids the best that we experience anxiety over every little detail of their development. And all that worry and stress can actually have the opposite effect of our intentions. Our kids are great, every one of them—gifted with their own unique talents and abilities—but those talents and abilities evolve over time. They don't need to be trained into a five-year-old. Our kids deserve every opportunity for greatness, yes, but they also deserve every opportunity to be raised in families that treasure and prioritize their childhood.

Relax. That's certainly what kids will do if you give them a chance. Most parents I know begin their parenting with a vow to not over-program their kids. But the crazy schedule kind of creeps up on us. We want our kids to be busy; we want them to learn, be active and meet friends. We set up play dates, we have piano on Monday night after school, on Wednesday there is soccer and on Friday swimming, and, of course, there's the soccer game on Saturday. In addition, there is homework to be done, and suddenly there is no time left over.

The alternative to over-programming our kids is

not the opposite—letting our children be idle. Rather, it involves balancing their structured time with their playtime, their time with instructors with their time with their family. I am suggesting that we look at our children's schedules and intentionally find time for family activities. We must find ways of being active together, and of letting our kids use their imaginations to create play. Early childhood is a particularly critical time for families to play together, and in our panic to give our kids a head start, many of us are missing out on a valuable experience.

Lessons and leagues *are* an incredible part of childhood. My ex-husband and I were both track athletes before we were rowers, and when we take our kids to watch a track meet we are flooded with strong and fantastic memories of our childhood clubs. "I just want them to have that much fun doing something," my ex said to me, "to experience some of the stuff I did as a kid." And there are lots of reasons to see organized sports as a positive part of your child's development. Playing on a team can build a child's self-esteem, teach them about teamwork, inspire them to set goals. It can also give children that precious feeling of accomplishment. Track was the only athletic commitment I had outside of school. I loved track, but it didn't prevent me from having time to play with my friends or to participate in school activities. We practised twice a week and had a meet every other weekend during the summer and a few each fall and winter. I tried to continue with my music lessons, but by the time I was fourteen I gave up piano because it was too much alongside track and school. Today, kids have track, piano, diving, tutoring and often races every weekend. I think it is out of balance. Every kid deserves some leisure time—time to use their imaginations, to find a friend and connect, to just play in their neighbourhood. In our efforts to give our kids every opportunity, I hope they don't miss the opportunity for a magical childhood.

Parents can fall into the trap of inadvertently pushing their children too hard. My son started competitive soccer eighteen months ago and has not scored a single goal, primarily because if anybody else is going after the ball, he is happy to give it to them. You can almost hear him saying, "It's okay, you take it." It is a bit maddening to watch, but on the other hand, isn't that what we have been instilling in him all along? Be kind, don't push, share. Suddenly when he is playing soccer he is supposed to elbow his way to the ball, take the ball from another player and be "aggressive"? I think his eight-year-old brain struggles with the contradictory messages. I think William will find his competitive instinct when he is ready; he will start to see that he can play aggressively but still be kind and considerate. I need to remind myself that he will discover his own motivation, his own competitive spirit, that my pushing him to be more aggressive will probably just make soccer less fun. On the other hand, my daughter scores goals almost by accident and has outstanding agility. However, the minute she perceives she is being watched or encouraged, she freezes and refuses to play. I guess the two make quite a team!

> Every kid deserves some leisure time—time to use their imaginations, to find a friend and connect, to just play in their neighbourhood.

I wonder why we as parents are in such a hurry. Do we want our kids to play adult games before they have had time to just have fun? Do we want to push them and get them to take on adult-like responsibility, to be competitive and motivated and hardworking, before they have even had time to be kids? No, of course we don't, but we need to step back and assess what kind of messages we are sending our kids with our actions and reactions. Let's give them the chance to enjoy just being a kid. As Rae Pica reminds us in her book *Your Active Child*, "childhood is not a dress rehearsal for adulthood."

One of the ways in which our children can enjoy activities that focus on having fun, learning new skills and making new friends is through our parks and recreation centres. I believe these centres are our country's best news when it comes to physical activity and community.

Glenn McLean, of the Canadian Parks and Recreation Association (CPRA), knows the number-one reason children choose to participate in sport: they are having fun. Keeping it fun involves offering a variety of programs, promoting inclusion, and challenging but not overwhelming kids with skill development. The programs aim to be affordable; in my rec centre, low-income families are given reduced admission. Nationally, a program called KidSport funds registration and equipment so *all* kids can play.

Until the age of ten, kids can't understand complex rules, strategies and coaching instructions. The coach may tell the kid to pass and go up the left wing, but when the whistle blows, the child just chases the ball. Young kids can focus on only one thing at a time, which means that if they are dribbling the ball it is unlikely it will even occur to them to pass it until a coach yells at them to do so. And then there is their distractability. We have all experienced it: my daughter was playing soccer last weekend and in the middle of the game, she stopped, looked up and noticed a bald eagle—no amount of coaching encouragement could get her focus back on the game (And how wonderful is it that she took the time to appreciate that bird's grace?)

That's not to say that kids should not be playing soccer at this age. Although they are not able to follow strategy and they don't entirely understand the rules, kids this age are developing their gross motor skills at a rapid rate. If they are in an organized league, it is important that skill development and fun are the main focus. This is an excellent time for them to grasp the fundamentals of games that include running, jumping and throwing. Having a good sense of the basics sets children up to enjoy a variety of sports as they get older.

Parents talk about young kids learning about teamwork, but kids younger than eight are egocentric. They lack the ability to put themselves in another person's position, or to truly work in a co-operative fashion.

Again, this doesn't mean that young kids shouldn't play sports, but I do think it means that our coaches have to understand children's developmental stages and shape their practise and game time to better reflect an understanding of that development. Having spent a year watching my son play in the local soccer league, I feel he gets significantly more exercise and skill development during the weekly practice than he does during games. Children at this age enjoy repetition, and younger players improve far more rapidly when allowed to practise a skill repeatedly. Of course, we all enjoy the games, but I certainly would like to see games played on a monthly basis and practices held a couple of times a week, so the coach could spend more time on skill development, fitness and fun. But it won't happen unless parents speak up. Increasing the ratio of practices to games goes against the conventional structure of most leagues. We should be rethinking this structure to allow for what's best for kids at different ages.

The right sport environment at the right time in a child's life can have a positive, transforming effect on that child's life. For many children, playing a sport is their first experience of being good at something. I remember this feeling well. I was the child who struggled in school—every subject required enormous effort, especially reading and writing. But at sports day in grade five, I won the half-mile run and came third in the high jump. This rare moment of being recognized for my abilities felt great, and it gave me a little bit of confidence in myself. Not surprisingly, as my confidence improved, my grades also began to improve. Now I can see the effect that such recognition has on my own kids. This year, for instance, my son's soccer coach gave every player on the team a certificate recognizing individual excellence. My son's certificate said "sharp shooter." For months after that, every time we would play soccer in the backyard, William would look at me and say, "Watch out, Mom, because I am the sharpest shooter!"

It is very important for young children to feel successful at a given task. According to Dr. Kenneth Cooper, who wrote *Fit Kids!* and started the Cooper Institute, a non-profit research and education centre that studies the relationships between living habits and health, kids under eight have trouble making the distinction between success or failure resulting from effort or training and success or failure resulting from lack of ability. They are likely to say "I am a bad goalie" when they let in a ball, rather than "I just need to practise being a goalie."

The right sport environment at the right time in a child's life can have a positive, transforming effect on that child's life.

When children are between the ages of nine and twelve, their bodies become highly receptive to training. This is a time when the body begins to develop much of its capacity for endurance and speed. The hours spent on a bike or time running down a soccer field or around a track build a level of fitness that sets a lifelong foundation. This is a good time to integrate physical, mental, cognitive and emotional components within a well-structured program. If fun is not a major component of their games, however, children this age will lose interest at what is a critical stage of skill and physical development. The trick is to get this age group doing a lot of running and jumping and throwing without them thinking they are "exercising." Almost every high-level athlete I know was extremely active in these formative years, often not in their chosen sports but in a variety of sports and play activities. Five-time Olympian sprinter Charmaine Crooks used to lift weights and run with her dad, which seemed like fun, not training. Olympic gold and silver medallist Derek Porter ran cross-country and played golf and soccer as a kid

Athletes who have trained in endurance sports at this age tend to have exceptional endurance later in their development; athletes who have focused on speed at this age tend to excel in speed sports later on. With this in mind, it makes sense to encourage children to play a wide variety of sports at this age—not only for fun, but to maximize their chances of doing really well in their favourite sport later in life. As parents and coaches, it is important that we focus our energy on giving children the components they need to do well in any chosen activity, and a positive experience that will lead to a positive feeling about sports.

For instance, training for speed and agility is

needed at this early age to ensure high performance down the road. Children at this age have short attention spans, so such training can be accomplished using chasing games, relays and beanbag races, all of which focus on speed and agility.

These stages are real and need to be considered, but they need to be considered in a far broader, more holistic approach to healthy children. It is even more important that we consider carefully whether our children are enjoying the activities they are involved in, whether they have adequate down time for outside play and interaction with their friends, and whether we as families have the amount of family time we desire. It doesn't have to be a choice between developing great athletes and having play and family time: the two can complement one another.

As we sign our kids up for sports there are some other elements worth considering. For example, who is the coach? Does he or she show true caring and understanding of children? At all ages, it is important that children get the "I care about you" message. Does the coach value fair play and equal play for all of the kids? Does the league have guidelines governing fair play and inclusion? Have the other parents committed to respecting officials, coaches and players? Shouting from the sidelines (as opposed to supportive cheering), over-competitive parents, and coaches who are too focused on winning can create negative experiences for young athletes, ones that could very well affect their lifelong relationships to sport. Sport is a great teacher for our children, and it is important that the sports we get involved in reflect the values we consider important.

Many people believe that sport has become too competition-based, that many professional athletes are not acting as appropriate role models and that parents' behaviour often ruins the experience for many kids. My experience in sports has been pretty positive, but when I attended a seminar about community sport called "The Sport We Want," I met several men and women who were absolutely opposed to competitive sport, whose own experience of being marginalized, bullied and pressured had embittered them to sport altogether. This is not what we want for our kids, but this has been the experience of many adults in sport, and it has led many people to fear competition for our kids in school, in sports and in recreation.

The seminar was hosted by True Sport, a national movement that passionately cares that the sport that exists in our communities is the sport we want—that it reflects what we value, what we hold dear about community sport. They are encouraging and supporting Canadians to look at community sport and ask, "Does what exists reflect my values?" Canadians believe that sport has enormous potential to teach our kids values like fair play, teamwork, goal setting and community caring, and yet 80% of Canadians surveyed believe that sport is not fulfilling its potential to positively influence our kids.

The belief in the extraordinary positive potential of sport to shape character and communities is the inspiration for True Sport. Ric Young, the architect of True Sport, has worked with the Canadian Centre for Ethics in Sport to create a movement focused on reintroducing "the sport we want." Says Victor LaChance of the CCES:

> Sport is a human construct; we have built it to be a certain way. It is built on certain principles and values; if we use golf as an example, the purpose is to take a ball and put it in a hole. All right, give me a ball and I'll drop it in the hole and the job's done. But that is not what's done—you give me a funny stick, you put the hole three hundred yards away, you put sand, trees and water in the way and say, "Now put the ball in the hole!" Why do we do that? We've made something extremely simple and straightforward hugely complicated! And it gives me

no greater gain . . . but that is the point. We've constructed it that way because it does give us something that we want: what we want is to be able to challenge ourselves. We want to work at the mastery of skills; we want to test ourselves against ourselves and others; we want to set goals and achieve them; we want to do things because they're difficult.

This is part of human nature. We have built sport around fundamental principles of fairness and contest: you aren't allowed to just pick up the ball and drop it into the hole. That to us is "true sport," and the people at the CCES and True Sport have worked with communities across this country to discover that this is the sport that people want—sport that is fair, that challenges our kids, that teaches them about themselves and others, that helps them be better.

If we think that sport should bring joy, we should seek to create sport in our communities that is joyful for children.

North Americans are passionate about sport. We remember our childhoods playing hockey and basketball; we mark the changing of the seasons by what sports we play, what jerseys we put on; adults throughout this country can be heard passionately debating last night's game; we watch the Olympics and feel pride in our athletes because we feel they represent the best that we can be and that our country can be. During the Olympic Games in 2000 in Sydney, when Daniel Igali won the gold for wrestling, I cried as he laid our flag down and kissed it. I actually sobbed, "He chose Canada. He chose *Canada*," when this Nigerian-born athlete received his medal. The sport that we create in our communities should reflect our values as a society. If we value fair competition and inclusion, our sport should reflect these values. If we think that sport should bring joy, we should seek to create sport in our communities that is joyful for children.

Minor hockey is infamous for its poor standards of sportsmanship from players, parents, officials and coaches. It seems that almost everybody has a story of parents screaming abuse at referees, parents getting into fights in the arena and players who take on the role of eliminators. In Nova Scotia, the Dartmouth Whalers Minor Hockey Association decided to create an environment that would give children happy memories of hockey. Spectators criticizing referees, abuse being hurled at players and coaches not giving weaker players ice time were part of the culture of minor hockey that the Dartmouth Whalers

Association wanted to put behind them. Executive members of the DWHMA developed a program called Fair Play, focused on making the sport of hockey a positive experience for children. They displayed banners and signs in arenas to advertise and educate participants about the program, they created a new process for selecting coaches and they asked each player, coach and parent to sign a contract outlining the rights, responsibilities and obligations of players, coaches and parents.

Sport needs be suited to each stage of a child's development, it needs to keep the child challenged and interested, and it needs to be fun.

Initially, the DWMHA was the only association with a Fair Play promotion program, but within two years the program had spread throughout the league. The effects of the program exceeded the creators' expectations. Suspensions in the league dropped 40%, referees and coaches stayed in their positions for longer terms, and the performance of the league improved dramatically. Minor hockey is flourishing in Dartmouth again.

This is the kind of positive culture in sport that True Sport is beginning to bring about throughout the country.

—

There are a few common themes running through all the stages of a child's development in sports. Sport needs be suited to each stage of a child's development, it needs to keep the child challenged and interested, and it needs to be fun.

As parents we have an important role in asking for the sport we want in our communities, asking that coaches care about children as people as well as as athletes, asking that sport be fun and fair and inclusive. I hope that those parents who had terribly negative experiences with sport as a child will make the effort to help create the sport they want for their kids and communities rather than deny their kids the unique gifts that a great sporting experience can give children. Through sport, kids can learn about effort translating into results, about working together for a desired result, about sharing success and setbacks, and about respecting their opponent. These are lessons that last a lifetime. Excellence and fun *can* go together. The fun factor needs to be part of the sport experience at every level. As an Olympic athlete, I can say that when the fun factor receded too far into the background, my performance suffered. Without fun and joy, we lose

Sport could and should give every child a place to have fun, to be included, to learn about values like teamwork and healthy competition.

the desire to work hard, compete and win. My mother's parting words every time I left for track practice—"Have fun and don't overdo it"—seem to increase in wisdom as I raise my own children.

Sport could and should give every child a place to have fun, to be included, to learn about values like teamwork and healthy competition, and to help that child aspire to their own personal excellence. This is what most of us want for our kids in their sporting experience, and it is what we all have the ability to be part of in our communities. Sport can be one of the very best memories of childhood and a positive part of raising healthy kids.

Why Children Play Sports

1. To have fun

2. To learn and improve skills

3. To be with friends and make new ones

4. For the excitement

5. To succeed or win

6. To exercise and become physically fit

Why Children Drop Out of Sports

1. Not enough playing time

2. Being criticised or insulted

3. Mismatching (ability and challenge)

4. Stress

5. Failure

6. Poor organization

Adapted from Canadian Parks and Recreation resource
Stephen J. Bavolek, Ph.D
National Institute for Child-Centered Coaching, Utah

"Now I'm the activist kid in the whole school!"

ACTION SCHOOLS! BC STUDENT

ACTIVE SCHOOLS

Seven million children in Canada spend seven and half hours each day in school. As families we can create active environments, but schools must provide opportunities for our kids to be active enough to achieve optimal health. And for those children whose parents are unable or unwilling to give their kids the physical activity their bodies require, school is the place where they should at least be guaranteed the minimum exercise required for good development. As parents, we need to care about what's going on when our kids are not under our careful eye.

Today we know so much about how a child

CHILD'S PLAY

learns and what a child needs. We know that children who are hungry can't concentrate, so volunteers and corporations have responded by providing breakfast programs. Both Kellogg's and McDonald's support breakfast programs that bring fresh fruit, hot cereal, eggs and toast to kids in inner-city schools. A provincial government grant through the "Students Success" program enables Nelson Mandela school in Toronto to provide a nutritious breakfast for kids. When children start their day with a healthy breakfast, they can focus on their studies rather than on their grumbling tummies. We also know that children who are not safe at home will have trouble reaching their academic potential. Increasingly, there are ways of identifying children who need extra support and giving them the interventions they need.

Current approaches to what gets included in and excluded from the curriculum and how teachers are trained do not reflect a passion for or a commitment to teaching the whole child. Children's intellects cannot be developed separately from their well-being, their physical health and their psychological state. We put enormous emphasis on academic achievement and allow physical activity and training to fall victim to budget cuts, lack of properly trained PE teachers and scheduling. By making our children's bodies less important than their minds, we are creating all kinds of problems and challenges—not only for their well-being, but for their attitudes toward school and learning.

Physical education was not my favourite subject. I hated having to change into those stupid bloomers, and when the bloomers finally disappeared there were those ugly polyester shorts. I dreaded baseball because I was completely hopeless at it. I would stand in the outfield and break into a cold sweat every time a batter was up, praying, "Please don't hit the ball my way." Now that I think about it, every subject at school had elements that alternately challenged, irritated, bored or terrified me. But somehow, my memories of gym are more visceral and hence longer-lasting. I remember the entire climbing apparatus shaking as I attempted to master the flexed-arm hang. I can still feel the bottom uneven bar banging against my stomach. There was simply no way to adjust the bars to adapt to a grade nine girl who was five foot ten.

I was a child who was easily embarrassed and stressed by new situations. In PE I experienced embarrassment at my lack of skill in sports, and stress when trying sports and skills that were new to me. The really

When children start their day with a healthy breakfast, they can focus on their studies rather than on their grumbling tummies.

good teachers assured me that I was not the only one who didn't know how to throw a baseball, and as an adult I realize that my lack of skill was more perceived than real. But in my child's brain, I was klutzy, awkward and uncoordinated. I am glad, however, that we had high-quality physical education taught four times a week at my school. With time I became more confident, and began to excel in some areas—though I remained markedly awful at gymnastics and dance. Having PE almost every day kept me healthy and pushed me to overcome my shyness and embarrassment.

I have spoken to many successful recreational athletes who dreaded the forty-minute gym class, who simply could not keep up with the jocks, who felt uncoordinated and vulnerable, who stressed about one or more of the activities even if they were athletic. I didn't love all of it either, but I am certain now that my body needed it—that spending forty minutes a day running, learning to throw a ball or choreographing a dance routine laid a foundation for many of the sports and activities I enjoy today.

In schools back then, there were also lots of opportunities to be active outside of gym class. Recess was an integral and fun part of my experience, and it was during that time that I gained my social skills and some of my confidence with parents and teachers. Similarly, playing a team sport was a major part of being in public school. We had baseball and track and basketball and the swim club. I was too shy to try out for team sports, but I got roped into one or two nonetheless. It was hard to do nothing: there were so many opportunities, and teachers went out of their way to get every kid involved in something. I didn't excel at any sport other than running, but I was still encouraged enough to play on teams. And who can forget the Canada Fitness Awards and ParticipAction, which got millions of schoolchildren running the 50-yard dash, sprinting between pylons and shaking so hard in an attempt to do 60 seconds of flexed-arm hang that the entire apparatus vibrated?

I remember my grade two teacher pointing to the vowels on the board, and me having no concept that these letters and sounds were building blocks of language. I was asked to repeat grade two, which did nothing to improve my belief that I was stupid. But what lessened the blow was the compassion and caring my teacher, Mrs. Finlayson, showed when she came to my house to give me the news (with a box of chocolates) and told me not to be too upset. She reminded me that everybody learns differently and that "everybody is good at something."

Two years later, another teacher at the school put up a poster inviting students to be part of the five-hundred-mile club. She chalked out the perimeter of our schoolyard and gave us sheets to use to keep track of how much we ran or walked—the goal was to walk five hundred miles within four months. The first day I walked four times around the perimeter, and by the end of the week I had logged six miles. I realized I was going to have to up the ante if I was going to meet the goal, so I began to walk-run, which was more fun than walking anyhow. Soon I was running the loop of the school dur-

> Every child deserves to feel good about him- or herself and to be given the opportunity to explore talents in sports, art, music and drama.

ing lunch hour and doing a few laps before and after school. Four months later, we had an assembly recognizing all the members of the running club. I was given a badge for completing 320 miles and congratulated in front of the whole school. It was the first time I had been recognized in an assembly or at school and it felt great. As an added bonus, I had become quite an enthusiastic runner.

I felt I was pretty good at running, and that belief improved my confidence and started to positively affect how much I enjoyed school. By the end of grade six I was one of the keenest readers in class, I was part of the basketball team and I would even put up my hand once in a while when a teacher asked a question.

Not every child will excel in academics, but every child deserves to feel good about him- or herself and to be given the opportunity to explore talents in sports, art, music and drama.

What strikes us as parents as our own kids enter grade school is that things have changed. Whether through budget cuts, increased focus on academic scoring, or the introduction of mega-schools where one gym serves more than a thousand kids, it's clear: priorities have shifted. At most elementary schools, after-school sports—if they exist at all—are sporadic and rely heavily on parent volunteers, and daily physical education, or even thrice-weekly hour-long gym time, is almost unheard of.

But the most shocking thing I have learned about physical activity in schools is that most elementary schools do not have a dedicated physical education teacher. This means that your children might be fourteen before they have the benefit of a trained PE specialist! That is simply too late. In British Columbia, district physical education consultants used to support teachers by running workshops, sharing ideas and inspiring and mentoring young teachers. Twenty-five years ago, British Columbia had over eighty physical education consultants working to support our teachers in this crucial area; today we have zero. If governments truly want to make a difference in the health of our children, a good place to start would be to give us back what we had twenty-five years ago and restore funding to school districts to allow them to hire back physical education consultants. Right now, PEI is the only province in Canada with a PE specialist in every elementary school. Ministries of education across the country are beginning to mandate minimum daily physical activity levels, which is a good start, but we need teachers who know how to use that time in inclusive, exciting and varied ways. Without the necessary training, this won't happen and the gym equipment will stay locked away gathering dust because teachers are not qualified to use it. Parental pressure is the only way this will change; we must demand higher-quality physical education in our elementary schools.

Teachers are hobbled before they get out of the gates—the preparation our elementary school teachers receive in physical education is woefully inadequate. Many receive as little as six hours of physical education teacher training during a four- or five-year bachelor of education degree. The University of Victoria's Faculty of Education is unique in Canada in that it offers students a one-year course in teaching physical education. And it is the only school in Canada where teaching students must take a full credit in physical education.

Can you imagine how intimidating and frustrating it would be to teach a subject for which you had been given virtually no training? Imagine you've been assigned to teach grade three math, and yet you've received no training on the subject as it applies to that age group. Sure, you might be a math enthusiast, but does that make you capable of teaching math to young children? You would have the curriculum, but you wouldn't have an understanding of where the kids were developmentally, nor of how to teach them the subject in a way that enabled them to successfully learn.

In math or science or English, this is completely unacceptable to us. Parents would be calling meetings, talking to their administrators and generally raising a legitimate ruckus. Yet we have somehow allowed physical education to become de-prioritized.

How can you possibly make PE a fun and important part of a child's day without proper training and some real knowledge of why it is so important to a child's optimal growth and development? Again, many teachers in this country are simply not adequately trained to teach PE with the enthusiasm it deserves. I know that if I were a teacher it would be intimidating to teach something I wasn't qualified in or that I didn't have the resources for. Imagine all the skills needed to teach a child to play volleyball and then leading a classroom through a volleyball game following the rules, engaging the most reluctant participants and making it fun. Even co-operative games, ones that stress teamwork, need to be learned and perfected through trial and error.

Running and jumping and throwing in gym class is not just a chance to blow off steam and be silly; gym helps children develop skills that become the foundation for a positive experience in movement and sports for the rest of their lives.

I have participated in workshops hosted by the Ontario Physical and Health Education Association (OPHEA) in which teachers learn how to play co-operative games and teach basic gymnastic skills. Training our teachers is not an enormous or onerous task. In one workshop I took in Fort McMurray, Alberta, called Motivating the Masses, I watched as elementary school teachers—most of whom were not physical education specialists—added to and suggested different versions of games before the session had even ended. I saw how their remarkable talent and enthusiasm for teaching kids improved within a single workshop. I was still trying to remember the games the instructor had described, and there they were inventing new ones! I only hoped that their principals and colleagues would support their enthusiasm once they returned to their schools.

Running and jumping and throwing in gym class is not just a chance to blow off steam and be silly; gym helps children develop skills that become the foundation for a positive experience in movement and sports for the rest of their lives. However, when children undergo formal instruction to develop skills and a positive attitude toward movement, they are too often instructed by teachers who are not empowered to give them a great experience in gym class. And if kids don't have a positive experience in gym in elementary school, they won't sign up for it in high school, often believing they are not good at sports or that they don't enjoy physical activity. Sadly, these attitudes can last a lifetime.

I tried to teach some grade one girls to do Chinese skipping (remember the elastic around two sets of ankles?) the other day and I was shocked to realize I had forgotten how to play. I felt very frustrated that I couldn't teach these kids a really fun game and that I didn't remember any of the skipping songs I had sung so enthusiastically as a child. Teachers with little training in physical education must feel this way frequently, and this would certainly erode their enthusiasm.

I want my kids to learn a wide variety of activities from an enthusiastic and specialist PE teacher so that they move into high school eager to take gym, try out for teams and keep their bodies healthy. I want them to begin this physical education early on so it has time to develop into a passion or, at the very least, into a natural and integral part of their lives.

Steve Friesen, the high school teacher I mentioned earlier, is the head of the health, physical education and athletics department at St. James Catholic High School in Guelph, Ontario. He says he can quickly tell whether a child has had a good physical education program in elementary school. If the kids are not participating at all in class, "It is a pretty good guess that their elementary school didn't do a lot to create a positive experience with physical activity. By grade nine a lot of them are already turned off PE." Steve and many others believe that if kids find sports and activities that excite them in high school, they are far more likely to be active as adults. And when they are active in high school, kids are active in the most critical time of their bone development. It is in the early teen years that children acquire 23% of their bone mass. Let it be volleyball or soccer or dance or fitness training—absolutely anything to get these early teens moving their bodies and loading their bones. We need to understand that gym isn't a luxury; it is a time when kids are strengthening their bodies, developing motor skills and building the attitudes and habits that can lead to lifelong well-being. It is a time for them to learn true teamwork and leadership; it is a chance to get to know their classmates in a dynamic setting. It's a time for kids to see that play and sport should follow them through their lives. And what would be better for that than an excited, creative and supportive (and supported!) PE teacher?

It is a ridiculous predicament for teachers and a bad-news story for our kids. It takes confidence and energy to lead kids in games and engage them in a physical activity. Confidence for teachers comes in the form of adequate training, familiarity with the subject, and good leadership. In addition to those challenges, teachers are overloaded by the diversity of the subjects they are supposed to teach, the time they need to teach each subject well and the number of children in their classrooms. It is easy to see how physical education and sports and outdoor time have been squeezed out of the equation.

A passionate desire to uncover the full potential of the child is what every great teacher has in common. "Every child is special," "Every child has a unique ability" and "All children can be good at something" are common refrains you hear from dedicated, compassionate teachers. We all have great teachers we remember, and their influence can affect us in unexpected ways. I got a letter from my camp counsellor not too long ago:

Thirty-four years ago a very delicate little girl with cornflower blue eyes and flaxen white hair came to Camp Totordeca in a lilac dress with a white cardigan, white patent leather shoes and frilly white socks. I thought to myself, "What a ridiculous outfit that little girl is wearing to an outdoor adventure camp." I sent her home that night looking like Pigpen, and she returned the next day wearing exactly the same outfit, only it was spotless! I remember thinking that the girl's mother must be crazy, but now I know it was the determination of her five-year-old daughter that allowed her to wear that same outfit every day.

As I read this letter now, I remember that little girl. Painfully timid, delicate and—frilly. I can remember those socks as if they were still in my drawer, and my insistence on wearing this beautiful outfit every day—all summer. How that little girl who wouldn't have said boo to anybody became a woman who strode onto the stage at the Mississauga Living Arts Centre this fall and spent an hour laughing and inspiring twelve hundred people about physical activity and our kids I am not quite sure. I suspect that many great teachers and coaches and abundant physical activity had a lot to do with the transformation.

The teachers I know want to help children discover their own excellence. They read books about teaching in their spare time (just as we pore over parenting books); they are fascinated by child development and speak to colleagues and leaders in the field to glean insight into their own teaching abilities. Get a good teacher talking about how a child learns and you had better have several hours free to engage in a lively discussion.

The subject that seems to be the exception to this rule is physical education. Teachers start off their careers with no tools for how to engage children in play and games. I have been told by several elementary school teachers how ill-equipped they feel to teach PE. They dread the class because they simply don't know what to do with the kids.

"People say how good kids have it these days. I'm thinking how bad they have it. I don't think things have gotten better; they've gotten worse because we've locked them in," says Steve Friesen. By "locking them in," he is referring to our reluctance to let kids play in the schoolyard after the school day is over. It is important for us all to remember that physical education is only one of many opportunities within the school day for kids to be active. In addition to PE, kids have recess time, lunch break, active classrooms, after-school games, intramural sports (teams that play purely within the school) and regular school teams (that compete with other schools).

Perhaps one of the greatest opportunities to get kids active is to use those moments within the school day when the kids are restless or lethargic to create opportunities to play, dance or get some fresh air. On a beautiful sunny day, my grade six math teacher used to teach math by getting us to measure the circumference of the playing field, to count bugs and create math equations, or to calculate the distance a student travelled using a pedometer. Parents need to support teachers' desire to be creative in getting kids moving. My friend Carla Pace, a teacher, says that in her elementary school some parents check to see how much time kids are playing outside and then accuse the teacher of not teaching during this time. Clearly, we all need to educate ourselves on the importance of movement for our children.

Fortunately, there are teachers out there who are transforming physical activity in their schools. They are not looking just to produce winning teams; they are looking to create an environment that encourages all kids to play. Steve Friesen worked with other teachers to completely transform the look and feel of physical activity in his school. Eight years ago, his school had only the traditional sports: football, basketball, volleyball. The vast majority of students didn't play after-school sports and dropped out of gym when it was no longer mandatory. Just three years later, more than 65% of students play intramural sports and there has been a huge increase in kids electing to take PE.

Friesen and his small group of teachers presented new ideas to the administration and had to fight hard to have changes brought in. Their goal was simple: they wanted to give every student a positive experience in physical activity. And their efforts have been successful. The athletic department now emphasizes participation, not just winning teams. Steve says, "In my mind, intramurals are just as important as football. Whether a child is a star football player or has little confidence in their athletic abilities, they are all kids and they are all getting active." Students form their own teams and the school even funds team T-shirts for each group. There are grad awards for intramurals, recognizing spirit, participation and excellence.

With their philosophy of 100% participation, Steve and his colleagues hope to turn all kids on to physical activity. Whether it's their gym designed more like a fitness facility, intramurals, after-school yoga classes or outdoor orienteering excursions, these teachers are creating excellence in the area of physical activity—excellence as measured in kids' enthusiasm for gym and after-school activities, excellence in terms of kids' attitudes toward school, excellence in capturing the imaginations of teenagers. As Steve says, "We have to connect what we do with the real world outside of us. I won't do any exercise I don't enjoy—it has to be fun or we won't stick with it. As long as it is fun, you are going to reach kids."

Elaine Devlin, who teaches grades seven and eight in Lakefield, Ontario, has helped create a school environment in which 80% of the kids play intramurals. Elaine has learned to get creative with intramural activities. From scooter hockey to dodge ball to Ultimate Frisbee, she imposes few rules about what can or can't be played. "What I try to do," she explains, "is to find some games that are different and interesting to the kids, and I take some time in class to teach the games and encourage students. A lot of times it's asking the kids what they're interested in. After the movie *Dodgeball* came out, dodge ball became the thing to do. So we developed rules based on our gym. Kids are pretty good at coming up with ideas, and when kids help create the rules, they are more willing to participate."

> Kids are the experts on play, not us, and we need to encourage them to play how *they* want to play, not how *we* want them to play.

I have discovered the same thing while playing with groups of kids in my neighbourhood: I teach them the game, and they create their own version of it. When children are allowed to determine how and what they play, when we allow their games to unfold in an organic manner according to how those particular kids on that particular night want to play, we are virtually guaranteed full participation and maximum enjoyment. Kids are the experts on play, not us, and we need to encourage them to play how *they* want to play, not how *we* want them to play.

Dr. Martin Collis is a world-renowned speaker on wellness, a retired professor of physical education and a former high school teacher. As a teacher, he had another interesting approach to involving his students: "What influenced my selection of activities in high school were activities that kids would pay to do out of school. When I saw that kids were paying to do aerobics classes, martial arts and Pilates, I created opportunities for these activities to happen within the school setting."

Finding something that everybody enjoys is important. At my son's school, a group of parents created a semi-organized play program called Games on the Green. We have taken most of the year to discover what games work and include the entire group, and what games only encourage the strong runners or the kids with exceptional hand-eye coordination. The art of teaching and coaching involves understanding the group you are leading and adapting activities to suit individual preferences and unique needs. Elaine has found scooter hockey—played sitting on scooter boards and using miniature hockey sticks—to be a great equalizer for kids with different levels of experience in hockey. No one at her school had played scooter hockey before, so everyone started at square one and felt comfortable participating. Steve Friesen finds wall-climbing a great equalizing activity. Creating a fun, welcoming and interactive environment for kids of all athletic abilities has been fundamental to Elaine's success with getting more kids out moving more often.

When asked how physical activity benefits the children in her school, Elaine responded,

> It gives them a chance to burn off steam and redirect the restlessness that builds up sitting through lessons. For me, and this is a big one, it allows kids the opportunity to play; my whole thing is to teach kids that it is okay to play and that everybody plays—even adults!—and when we play we have fun. I think the image of play we have now has affected our youth. We believe that only little kids should play

and as a result, a lot of us don't know how to play anymore. We don't know how to create our own games.

I think it is so sad that we have raised a generation of kids who think it is not cool to play. Maybe we have forced them to be too serious, too "mature." Maybe they need to see adults running and yelling and jumping, laughing and having fun, in order to feel that it's okay to just want to play.

In our culture, playfulness is often equated with childishness. Yet nurturing playfulness in children and in adults leads to an increased joy for life and balances the pressures and responsibilities of life. The best thing I can do after a hectic day in the office is to go outside and play a game of tag with my son, or pick up a piece of sidewalk chalk and draw a picture on the driveway with my daughter.

Teaching games is important to Elaine, important enough to organize her students' field trip during the coldest time of the year. Why? "Because there's nothing to do," she laughed, "so the trip becomes a great thing to do!" Rather than planning class trips to Ottawa or Kingston, Elaine takes her students to an outdoor centre. After dinner each night, the kids put on all their gear and go outside to play a version of capture-the-flag they have developed over the years, called "Survival." "We play for hours," Elaine told me, "and the kids don't even realize how long they've been out!" One of Elaine's most treasured memories is of one group that loved playing Survival so much that they continued to meet every Friday night to play until the end of the school year. "They took to that whole idea that you can be in grade seven or eight and still play," Elaine said, "and I think that is pretty cool."

Teachers like Steve and Elaine show us what is possible with passion, creativity and a belief that change is possible. Not every teacher has this kind of commitment to getting kids healthy. It is unfortunate that it requires so much energy and tenacity to create healthy, active environments for our children to learn in.

In the national report card on children's health done by Active Healthy Kids Canada that I mentioned earlier, our schools were given an F in daily physical education, because only 14% of them provide the recommended 150 minutes of physical education each week. Our schools were given a D– in trained physical education personnel. To put this in perspective, as fitness advocate Tim Lane reminded me, there are even guidelines that govern how much daily activity a chicken needs to be considered "free-range." We need more free-range kids!

Obviously, we can't just assume that educators know how unhealthy our children are. When I spoke to eight hundred teachers at an education conference in Peterborough, Ontario, it was clear that all of them had the well-being of children first and foremost in their minds, but many admitted to forgetting or to not realizing the importance of physical activity as a integral part of a good education. Schools have been so focused on academics that teachers often judge their own performances by how well the kids do academically. While parents and educators graph grade-school averages, subjects like physical education, music and art have been relegated to the category of "extras." While in Peterborough, I spoke to senior administrators for the Kawartha Pine Ridge school district about creating more opportunities for kids to be active in their schools. When I talked about kids enjoying school more and concentrating better and about the schools' responsibility for helping our kids be physically and spiritually well again, the educators were listening. Having the opportunity to sit in a small group and talk about the value of physical activity in our schools gave them a chance to really reflect on their role in producing healthy kids. The board committed to an additional twenty minutes of physical activity a day. Wow.

According to Dr. Collis, one Vancouver high

school used to keep something called a SPARC (student physical activity record card) for each student. The card featured information on strength, endurance, flexibility and other measures of fitness. The SPARC was presented to students along with their graduation certificates. This is the type of report card that can help parents understand how their children are progressing physically and to alert them to potential problems. If the health or ill health of our children was spelled out in black and white terms, it would be more difficult to ignore our responsibilities. As parents we can work with our parent councils to evaluate physical activity in our schools. A good place to start is with the Quality Daily Physical Education (QDPE) Report Card, which is available at www.cahperd.ca. Fill it out and see how your school is doing.

> While parents and educators graph grade-school averages, subjects like physical education, music and art have been relegated to the category of "extras."

Thankfully, awareness of the critical importance of physical activity in our schools is on the rise. Governments are beginning to understand the link between inactive kids and unhealthy adults. In

September 2005, both Ontario and Alberta implemented the Daily Physical Activity Initiative, which mandates thirty minutes of daily physical activity for all students in grades one through nine. This is a great program in theory, but mandatory quantity requirements without also looking at quality could prove counterproductive. Teachers can't be expected to suddenly find the tools to make kids more active. That takes leadership, training and funding. Somebody has got to be leading workshops, providing teaching resources, increasing budgets and having experts visit the schools to share their knowledge and enthusiasm. When you provide information and tools and you back them up with a strong commitment within the administration, teachers will do remarkably creative and innovative things to get kids moving.

Schools that have made a concerted effort to focus on creating an active school environment regularly hear back from parents about how much their kids are enjoying school.

Colin Inglis of the City Centre Education Project (CCEP) in Edmonton knows how to be innovative. He brought together seven inner-city schools to share resources, and developed a strategy to enrich the schooling and improve the health of students. Kids had the opportunity to be picked up from school and to be enrolled in YMCA programs, and got access to counselling services and healthy food in school. Colin's belief is that all kids need the same things to excel in school and life and that "what is good for the best is good for the rest." If there aren't resources in the family to provide these advantages, then they have to come from somewhere else. He even brought in personal trainers for the most reluctant teenage girls, who apparently responded well to PE when they were treated like "movie stars." These girls quickly came to love their yoga, Pilates and hip-hop dance sessions and stayed active during the most critical stage of their bone development. Of course, they weren't thinking of bone development—they were feeling special and having fun. This group of schools in Edmonton illustrates to all of us that change is not only possible, it is already happening.

It is difficult to be passionate about something you don't fully understand the value of, and it's nearly impossible to make a difference when you feel as if you're the only one who cares. Many of the administrators and teachers I have interviewed for this book do not fully realize the benefits of a physically active school. And more often than not, the ones who do recognize it feel powerless to change things. Just as I have argued for educating the whole child, so I am arguing for a "whole" education system.

Schools that have made a concerted effort to focus on creating an active school environment regularly hear back from parents about how much their kids are enjoying school. Lunch runs, lunch-hour sports and active schoolyard play are all terrific ways of building school spirit and kids' sense of belonging. Research confirms that daily physical education contributes to the health and fitness of children and also improves children's attitudes toward and enjoyment of school. A study conducted by the California Department of Education in 2002 of nearly a million schoolchildren clearly demonstrated the connection between physical activity and improved academic performance. The study looked at six measures of fitness for schoolchildren in grades five, seven and nine. It also used standardized tests to measure their performance in mathematics and reading. In simple terms, the results showed that the fitter the child, the better the academic performance. As fitness levels increased, so did academic scores. Whatever the grade level and whatever the gender, the higher the fitness scores, the better the scores were in math and reading.

Here in Canada, the Action Schools! BC pilot project studied five hundred elementary school students and measured blood lipid levels, bone density and cardiovascular fitness as well as academic performance and attitudes toward school. Although this pilot study was unable to directly link improved academic performance to increased physical activity, what *was* clear was that children's attitudes toward school became markedly more positive when more physical activity was introduced. Since then, the Action Schools! BC program has spread province-wide, helping schools create plans to get kids moving—in their classrooms and playgrounds as well as during gym time. Today, more than six hundred schools are registered as Action Schools. Children in Action Schools can be found bouncing at the bell, hip-hopping to music for the ten minutes between math and English, taking geography class outdoors or going for a thirty-minute walk upon arrival each morning. Don't believe me? In Saskatoon thirty-five thousand schoolchildren start their day with a community walk (initiated by Saskatoon in Motion). They walk in the dead of winter and the kids love it! They also focus more energy on nationwide fitness initiatives such as Jump Rope for Heart and the Terry Fox Run.

When we allow our schools to use teachers with no training, the implicit message is clear: physical education is not important. This sends a dangerous message to our kids: your physical health is not important. If parents, teachers and principals don't value physical activity, why should kids? The most powerful action a teacher can take is to put on her own running shoes and enthusiastically participate in activities. William became skilled and enthusiastic about skipping not because I spent hours with him in our driveway calling "Jump, jump," (which I did, with no success), but because his kindergarten teacher, Mrs. Metters, was an enthusiastic believer that kids should move and managed to get every kid in her class skipping and singing skipping songs. She is a great example of somebody who took it upon herself to create an outstanding physical education experience for the kids she taught.

My friend Carla Pace says, "I think that the teachers who get their kids really active are willing to bend the rules a little bit, to take them outside during art class, to find a window of time in the afternoon to play soccer." Two years ago, she found herself teaching a grade three class with twenty-two boys and eight girls. The energy in the class was driving her nuts, so she began to take the kids outside every afternoon for a half-hour game of soccer. "I noticed a marked increase in their concentration after the game," she says, "and an increased motivation to finish the work so they could get outside and play." As parents we know this is true: when sibling rivalry leads to hitting and the energy in the room is getting too frantic, we tell our kids to "take it outside." Teachers should take the opportunity to do the same thing with the kids in their classroom—to get creative, to meet the challenge of getting kids active in the school setting, to take an idea or a resource and make it their own.

Let's go back to that math example. Imagine if, in the elementary school your child attended, no teacher had formal training in teaching math. Then imagine that the school principal didn't particularly value math so she didn't hire experts in math and math received only limited funding. In that school, your child would not have the opportunity to realize his full potential in the subject of math. Well, this is exactly the fitness environment that exists in most of the public schools in North America. Physical education is treated like something that is nice to have but not particularly needed. We *must* rethink our priorities and raise a ruckus on behalf of our kids' health. We *must* talk to our principals and school administrators about how important physical education is to the teaching of our children. We *must* support our schools when they introduce healthy food policies and when they take time during the school day to allow our kids to be active.

As parents you have the power to influence change. Demand the funding from politicians for physical education consultants; find out about the quality of PE at your child's school; have your parent council fill in a QDPE Report Card; and let the principal and the teachers know that you value your child's health and development and would like to see PE workshops and intramurals at the school and teachers enrolled in PE courses on professional development days.

Even when we do have dedicated physical education teachers, we disempower them by shortening gym classes to between twenty and forty minutes. Children have hardly enough time to change into shorts and runners before the bell rings signalling the next subject. (In fact, most elementary schools no longer require children to have a gym kit—if your school doesn't require kids to be dressed for activity, how energetic can the lessons actually be?) We have often cut back teachers' budgets and restricted the activities they do teach. As Steve Friesen says, for math and science the red carpet is laid out, but if you want something in physical education, you have to make a strong case for change and be an advocate for the kids.

Many of us played on intramural teams during the lunch hour, were part of the running club or played on the school softball team. But organized sports are something of the past in most elementary schools today. In many districts, teachers are not paid for their after-school coaching time, and with the increased demands on their time in core subjects, they are simply not volunteering for after-school sports. In my children's school, all of the after-school sports are led by parents. It is great that parents are taking the initiative, but an enthusiastic and trained teacher should be involved in these types of school activities. The parent volunteers would then have someone within the school advocating for their needs—a teacher who knows and understands the kids—and would feel supported by the school in their initiative.

Recess is another great time for kids to be active. Our teachers never withheld recess. That was out of the question. We played outside, rain, snow or shine, because there was a basic, deeply held believe that fresh air and exercise were good for kids. In my entire public school life, I do not remember a single day that we did not go out to play.

I am deeply disturbed when I hear about kids missing recess because they didn't finish their math. This just reinforces the idea that recess is a special privilege instead of something kids *need* in order to be healthy and concentrate on their work. It screams to me, "We don't think physical activity is important!" And as for schools that have recess only in good weather, I can't help but wonder who doesn't want to go outside, the teachers or the students. I hear the excuse that kids don't have proper outdoor clothing, but I refuse to believe this is an insurmountable obstacle.

Teachers tell me that children today don't know how to play outside—that they get outside and just stand around. (Don't get me started on the "no running" rules!) Kids used to teach each other games like four-square, tetherball and marbles, but there has been a whole generation that hasn't learned to play schoolyard games. As a result, the games, the rules and the songs have often been lost.

Resources like *Positive Playgrounds*, which is a step-by-step manual that teaches volunteer parents and teachers how to create more active playgrounds, have successfully changed the landscape of many schools. Edmonton parent of two Pearl Marko developed *Positive Playgrounds* because she could not sit by and watch her children and their friends looking bored in the school playground. It was as if they had forgotten how to play. The games she remembered from childhood had not been passed on. Pearl field-tested 160 playground games and reproduced them in the manual to remind adults of the games and songs we enjoyed as children. It seems almost ridiculous that we need a guide to teach us how to help our kids play, but sometimes

> Kids want to play, they want to try new games, they enjoy running around . . . Sometimes adults just have to help them get started.

that is exactly what we need, and we shouldn't be embarrassed to admit it.

When her daughter Rhianna started kindergarten, my business manager Sandra Hamilton took it upon herself to show up at recess at her school once a week to teach the kids games, turn the skipping rope and sing the skipping songs. She wondered whether kids would be interested, but within a couple of days they were mobbing her the minute she arrived on the playground—girls *and* boys. Kids want to play, they want to try new games, they enjoy running around . . . Sometimes adults just have to help them get started.

Don Roberts's passion for healthy, active kids has spanned three decades. As a principal in the Yukon, he did a lot of research to confirm what he knew from experience. "If you are not creating a firm foundation of fitness and health in a child, you are not creating an environment for that child to reach his full potential as a human being," Don says. "Schools are supposed to have a child's entire well-being as a priority; they are truly charged with teaching to the whole child. In my years I have noticed that when kids have sufficient play and sports time, they approach their academics with more vigour. When teachers come to me and tell me their kids are misbehaving so they are going to cancel gym or recess, I tell them the reason they are misbehaving is because they are not active. If we allow teachers to cancel PE, we are sending out the message that it is not an important subject, that it is an 'extra.'"

Not only does Don convince the teachers and parents that PE and after-school sports are important, but he creates opportunities for the teachers to be successful. He brings in workshops to give his teachers the skills to teach PE, and for each of the schools he has been a principal for, he has been able to hire a full-time PE teacher, who not only teaches the kids but works with other teachers to improve their skills. "Sometimes," he says, "I will take teachers' math classes so they can teach PE—they know I am going the extra distance." All the teachers I have spoken with who have created great active programs in their schools stress the importance of a supportive administration. Doug Gleddie from Ever Active Schools in Alberta says that a supportive principal who understands the importance of physical education and of teaching to the whole child is the biggest determinant in how active and healthy a school will be.

When it comes to teaching the whole child, we have taken our eye off the ball. Our children have become more passive at school, less active during recess and less engaged in physical education. We have almost forgotten our children have bodies—and that their bodies are their primary way of experiencing the world. We have downloaded responsibility for PE to generalist teachers, and we have allowed gym class to become optional in high school. We have stood by and watched as sports have disappeared off the landscape of the school experience—intramurals are an archaic oddity—and playground time has been turned into something that may happen if we get through our work.

We need to do better. I believe an enormous cultural shift needs to take place in our schools. We must become vocal supporters of excellence in regards to our children's physical bodies. Our children have suffered not only physically, as I showed in the bad-news chapter of this book, but mentally and emotionally. We have to understand how the whole child has been affected, how fully our kids have been short-changed. I want my children to excel academically, but not at the cost of becoming stressed and unhealthy—not at the cost of being disengaged from their bodies and robbed of many of the joys of play and sports.

A supportive principal who understands the importance of physical education and teaching to the whole child is the biggest determinant in how active and healthy a school will be.

Of course, there are a lot of barriers to our kids' having daily physical education. When we are building mega-schools with fifteen hundred kids and one gym, even the most enthusiastic advocate of physical education will have a hard time getting every student a gym class. School boards need to understand the physical needs of children before schools are built. But even in these enormous schools, if physical activity is a priority, teachers will find ways to make it happen—teaching outside, getting kids more active in class or dividing the gym when necessary.

In British Columbia, Action Schools! BC master trainer and teacher Judy Howard has created a series of short videos called "Energy Blasts" that get kids dancing and moving in the classroom. In the United States, a company called Cool Zebra has created an educational hip-hop DVD about health that is fun and funky and engages kids. This resource will soon be available for a low cost to teachers throughout Canada. These are the kind of materials that are needed within every school so teachers have innovative ways to get their students moving. The adult fitness craze in the past two decades has created huge amounts of learning, resources and innovation. That innovation could be used in the classrooms and schools of this country.

Stephen Spencely, a teacher in Brampton, Ontario, endeavours to give each child in his school new experiences in activity. Stephen's school has a large population of new Canadians, many of whom have never worn a set of ice skates. But Mr. S., as he is affectionately known, owns four hundred pairs of skates, which he loans out to kids and families that need them. He found ways of getting every kid in the school skating or swimming or curling or even snow-boarding—activities they otherwise may not have had an opportunity to try—before they left elementary school. He even runs a school store that last year raised $37,000 to fund the kids' activities.

A teacher I know in Vancouver led her English class through stations in the schoolyard. Each station had a quiz about one of the Shakespeare plays they were studying, and the kids had to answer all of the questions before heading off as a team to find clues that would help them answer the final question. She tells me that the kids were running like crazy from station to station, combing the schoolyard at breakneck speed looking for clues. Best of all, nobody complained of being tired or that Shakespeare was boring. She has even had her kids do skits on the playground, or mini-productions of plays in the woods near the school.

If we work from the assumption that kids are naturally active, that they need to stay active to be healthy and to maximize their potential, we will find ways within our school environments to let them move. Let's give our teachers the skills and resources to do what they do best: take a little training and knowledge, then innovate and figure out how best to reach the child.

As a parent, I entrust my children to the school system for five full days a week. As I hand my little ones over, I pray that the teachers and schools educating my children will hold their minds, bodies and spirits in high esteem. I need to know that they will do the utmost to encourage in my children a love for learning, a connection to their physical bodies and a respect for their own unique spirits.

However, I will *not* remain passive to the process: I need to be clear about what I expect from the school and its teachers. I need to ask what's going on. I need to participate in making the school a healthier and more active place.

What You Can Do in Your Child's School

1. Ask how much physical activity your child is getting each day. Is the teacher trained to teach PE? If he or she is not a specialist PE teacher, when was the last time the teacher took a course on teaching PE?

2. Ask about the activities they are doing during gym class. Are they moving enough? Is there enough variety to engage everyone? How are reluctant students encouraged and included—or do they just sit out?

3. Let the principal know your child's health matters. Ask for a dedicated PE instructor, one who has received specific training in teaching physical education.

4. Ask about equipment: Are there enough skipping ropes, balls, etc., so that all of the children can participate?

5. Suggest that your school participate in an Action Schools program.

6   Talk to the principal about replacing junk food and pop machines with healthier options.

7. Volunteer to oversee a weekly after-school session of unstructured play.

8. Fill out the CAHPERD QDPE report card.

9. Engage the PAC (Parent Advisory Council) in making child health a priority of the school..

10. Tell your school trustee, MLA and MP that healthy, active schools are important to you, and that you want PE consultants rehired and elementary teachers trained to teach physical education.

"Everything that is good about communities, about schools, about individuals, young and old, is there for an afternoon."

TEACHER ROSS DAVIES SPEAKING
ABOUT THE TERRY FOX RUN

CHAMPIONS IN OUR COMMUNITIES

In one of the most isolated and northern communities in the Yukon, young Native people are building dreams, gaining self-esteem and learning life skills under the guidance of a Catholic priest from France. Father Jean-Marie Mouchet's classroom is not a church, but the wilderness surrounding the town of Old Crow. His lessons are not chapters of the Bible, but laps of the cross-country ski trails. For the kids who go through Father Mouchet's ski camp, the greatest teacher is their own minds and bodies working in concert with the natural beauty of the landscape. As the skiers challenge themselves on the steep hills and windy corners of the terrain, they learn about the power of using their bodies to commune with nature. They learn about the power of their own minds, and how to tap into it to overcome their burning leg muscles and the tightness in their chests. They learn that nature holds many lessons and adventures and promises, and they begin to see their strong bodies as the keys to accessing this world. As they start another lap of the five-kilometre trail, they grow more confident in themselves and their abilities: they begin to dream about possibility; they imagine a new role for themselves in their families and communities—all to the soundtrack of their pounding hearts and the cold squeak of snow.

For the kids who go through Father Mouchet's ski camp, the greatest teacher is their own minds and bodies working in concert with the natural beauty of the landscape.

Father Mouchet came to the settlement of Old Crow in 1954. When he arrived, he found that the community was already being serviced by an Anglican priest. Yet Father Mouchet was greatly affected by the raw and inspiring beauty of the land—and by the Gwich'in people, who were defined by their deep and ancient connection to it—so he decided to stay. Instead of trying to convert the population to

Catholicism, he would contribute in other ways. Determining that he needed to learn before he could teach, he chose first to be a student of that great and humbling place.

One of the first things Father Mouchet observed was that the community was in transition. The Gwich'in culture was undergoing a massive and profound shift, from a hunter-gatherer society to a more modern-style community. Families were moving off the land into town; children were attending church- and state-regulated schools. Hunting, previously the mainstay of the diet, became secondary to grocery stores full of packaged food and wilted produce. Many of the young people were losing their connection to the land and were living in unhealthy ways. Father Mouchet believed this put the young people of Old Crow at enormous risk for low self-esteem and a loss of purpose. He saw the culture's chance at survival as being in jeopardy because of the changes that were taking place, and he felt compelled to help in whatever ways he could.

He dedicated the next forty-seven years to the people of the North. In the twenty-five years he spent at Old Crow, he did not convert a single member of the community to the Catholic faith, a fact he is very proud of. Instead, his mission was to convert the people of Old Crow to a new lifestyle, one in which they would recognize their physical potential and use that potential to survive in the modern world. An avid outdoorsman and cross-country skier, Father Mouchet saw in the youth of Old Crow a natural disposition to move over snowscapes, a disposition they inherited from the physically challenging life their elders had led hunting and trapping, spending weeks at a time snowshoeing along their traplines. This lifestyle fed not only their bodies but their spirits and myths and legends. The ways of the Gwich'in elders held the stories of a culture, the great lessons of the past and an understanding of the people's place in the future. Their way of life was their breath, and this breath was slowly being suffocated out of them in the drive to modernize the North. The youth of Old Crow deserved to be proud of their culture and heritage; they deserved to have their country validate and encourage it; they deserved the relationship their elders and ancestors had with the land, and this relationship deserved to be protected and honoured. Father Mouchet saw cross-country skiing as an important way to help Gwich'in youth discover this connection—not only because he noticed their ability to move over snow, but because he knew what being intimate with nature had done for him in his own life, how the hard work of his body and the discipline of his mind elevated his confidence.

The move into the town, which was perhaps the most drastic change the Gwich'in had to deal with, would have an effect on everyone. Paul Andrews, a skier who went through Father Mouchet's program a few years later, when it had expanded to Inuvik, remembers starting at the town's school: "Here I was, out in the bush, and then suddenly I was in a town of four thousand people, and it was totally different. I didn't know what a gymnasium was, I didn't know what a big school was. I was terribly, terribly lost. The only time I would feel comfortable is when I was skiing out on the land. It felt like I was at home again, out hunting. If there was anything that preserved my sanity, it was Father Mouchet allowing me to be out on the land—without that I could have easily gone astray."

> Cross-country skiing soon became a focal point for the community. The entire town would show up for races, to cheer their children on and watch the young rising stars.

Father Mouchet began with just a few young people, most of whom had never skied before. The people of Old Crow had hunted and trapped on the land for generations and the kids were in great physical shape, but with the move into town, the physical outlet was gone.

He began by simply asking young people if they wanted to learn to ski. As kids learned, they began to tell others about it. For a short time Father Mouchet taught skiing in Faïrbanks at the army base, and he used the money he earned to buy ski equipment for the kids in Old Crow. His approach was to show by example, and he skied each day with the children. His passion for the sport and his deep caring for the children he coached were the primary reasons that within a few years, almost all of the kids in Old Crow were cross-country skiing.

Father Mouchet could be found skiing the trails with his fastest skier, or running behind his slowest skier, supporting, pushing, encouraging. In Old Crow, he managed to get the majority of the young kids aged six and up practising and competing. The young people were developing healthy bodies, but most importantly they were rebuilding their self-esteem. In that isolated place, where much of the community's sense of purpose had evaporated with their traditional lifestyles, cross-country skiing gave the kids dreams and goals, taught them the relationship between effort and reward, and allowed them to become part of something that had meaning.

Cross-country skiing soon became a focal point for the community. The entire town would show up for races, to cheer their children on and watch the young rising stars. The skiing became part of the social fabric, and it was common to hold get-togethers and celebrations to coincide with a cross-country race. As a lifetime friend of Father Mouchet's named Don Roberts told me, "If you talk to the seniors today in Old Crow, almost all of them took part in skiing in one form or another. It was a very strong program in the community when Father Mouchet lived in Old Crow, and the community was very proud of their youth who took part. Well over half of the youth during his stay in Old Crow took part in the ski program."

Father Mouchet was, and still is, an inspiring and outstanding coach, and when these young skiers began to compete outside of Old Crow, they won their share of medals. In 1963, Martha Benjamin, a twenty-five-year-old mother of five from Old Crow, stunned the ski world by winning the Canadian senior women's championships. When the Old Crow skiers won every event at the junior nationals a couple of years later, the world began to take notice. The government came on board with money to support the cross-country skiing, and in 1967 Father Mouchet founded the Territorial Experimental Ski Training (TEST) program. When Father Mouchet set up his program in larger communities—Inuvik and Whitehorse—the perception of this small town and its people began to change. The townspeople of Old

Crow took enormous pride in their skiers' accomplishments, and the skiers made quite a splash wherever they travelled. As one of the town residents said, "The mail run only used to go to Inuvik, but after we started winning big races, the mail stopped here. Skiing put this community on the map."

Sisters Sharon and Shirley Firth emerged as young stars through the TEST program in Inuvik. These two women are renowned throughout the Yukon; they became North American champions and competed in four Olympics. As the Firth sisters commented in Father Mouchet's book *Men and Women of the Tundra*, "Father Mouchet gave us the opportunity to prove to ourselves and the world that aboriginal people could excel in international competition."

Father Mouchet, with his TEST program, left a lasting legacy in the North, not only by producing world-class skiers, but by assisting hundreds of kids in developing good self-esteem and strong life and leadership skills. As Paul Andrews recalls, "He basically taught us, you know that hill, you could ski up that hill, and once you get up there, you'll have a nice slide down the other side. It's basically the same thing about life: you work hard, you go through all that 'it's hard and I don't want to do that,' and then it gets a little easier for a little while, you bask in the glory, and then another bigger hill comes along, but it doesn't seem like such a terrible hill once you've conquered the first hill. The point was not the skiing or the winning." Kids need to set goals and to experience success in order to build their self-esteem. Mastering new skills, setting a goal and meeting it, and experiencing commitment and caring from a respected member of the community can be instrumental to this development.

I met Father Mouchet a few years ago, while attending a Sport Yukon Awards dinner. He was in his early eighties and still struck me as charismatic and passionate. He remembered my race from the Olympics and complimented me as a "girl with a very strong mind!" As he returned to his seat at the dinner, I watched as everybody stood up to greet him, share a few kind words and shake his hand. In the Yukon, almost everybody has heard of Father Mouchet, and many Yukon residents have been through a TEST program themselves. In Victoria, I met a thirty-five-year-old woman named Janice who had been through the program in Whitehorse. She believes TEST and Father Mouchet had an enormous impact on who she is today: "The TEST program showed me that to see results you have to work hard; it taught me to be dedicated and self-disciplined." When I mentioned Father Mouchet her eyes lit up. She talked about how he had made her feel so important and special, and how he had shown her what she was capable of.

When Father Mouchet retired and left Old Crow, the program began to lose momentum. Since then, problems have begun to re-emerge in this northern Native community. Forty years after the inception of the skiing program, change is happening again: old cabins are being replaced by new houses, an airstrip cuts across the town, televisions with five hundred plus channels exist in virtually every home, and alcohol and urban street drugs have made their way into the lives of many people. The sense of isolation is less of a reality since planes come in every day, roaring down the ridiculously large airstrip, but the disconnection is there. Children are also becoming increasingly unhealthy, overweight and obese. As one elder said, "If we can't break the cycle for our young people, how do we keep going? All we can do is hope and pray for the younger generation. I look at what is here, and I have a lot of dreams for the younger generation and a lot of hope."

Today, Father Mouchet is once again part of rebuilding the TEST program in Old Crow, almost forty years after it started. The challenges in Old Crow may be different from when Father Mouchet first arrived, but his belief that sport can build self-esteem and inspire healthy choices in young people is still the fundamental principle behind the new initiative. So much success has been experienced in this little community, so many children's lives were transformed through sport—it would be tragic to see that legacy lost.

Through a series of magical coincidences, my dear school friend Jane Vincent and her partner, Trevor Browne, have been charged with revitalizing TEST in Old Crow. But Jane and Trevor have found that by only trying to recreate the TEST program they are connecting with too few young people. As a result, they have revamped the model and are now working inside the schools to take kids cross-country skiing during the lunch hour. This approach does not rely on parents to supervise kids, and it does not ask for a commitment from the children that they are not yet ready to make. Jane and Trevor have also taken several of the kids out winter camping, snowshoeing and on an overnight ski trip. Remarkably, for some of these kids, this was their first experience being out on the land overnight.

Father Mouchet and the people he inspired remind me once again that we have a deep longing to connect with one another. There is a hunger to move outside our homes, our places of work, our immediate relations—to connect with one another and care about one another. We seem to intuitively understand that the health of our neighbourhoods and our quality of life are deeply dependent on us working together. We want to live in communities where we care about our neighbours and where everyone shows an interest in investing in our collective future.

There are many people across this country who are transforming their communities one child, one initiative at a time. My girlfriend Laurie Anne is one of them. She walks her children to school almost every day and takes at least three more with her. She decided that the one-practice-to-one-game schedule of soccer didn't make sense for her five-year-old and for her family time, so she hired a soccer coach who wanted to teach the kids skills and let them play rather than have them compete in tournaments each weekend. This way the kids have lots of fun without cutting into weekend family time. She gets her exercise by volunteering once a week at the cycling club, where she pushes small children up really big hills. In her community, she often takes care of the kids whose moms and dads work late; she feeds a friend's child who she knows doesn't eat that well. In many little ways she is having a significant impact. Laurie Anne knows everyone, and her friends and community value her. I think she represents much of what we long for.

—

The greatest blessing that being a speaker and a high-profile Canadian has brought me is the opportunity to travel to almost every corner of this beautiful country. I have listened to the howling of coyotes from my room at a bed and breakfast in Grand Prairie; I have snowshoed through twenty feet of snow in Inuvik; I have sat in the shade in Winnipeg on a hot and sticky day; I have enjoyed a play in downtown Toronto. I am awed by the beauty of our landscape, the diversity of our cities and the passion most Canadians have for where they live. Whether I am sitting with a Winnipegger overflowing with excitement about the fringe theatre festival or listening to a Yukoner tell her story of dogsledding on the Yukon River, I am warmed by our love for where we live. Most Canadians would literally not want to live anywhere else than where they are living right now.

Sometimes I find this difficult to comprehend. As I leaned into the biting minus-thirty wind walking from my hotel room to the conference centre in downtown Winnipeg (definitely *not* a hot and sticky day!), I decided this was just some strong form of positive self-talk we all have. But listen to farmers in Saskatchewan or fishermen in PEI when they talk about where they live—they always begin their reveries saying, "The people here are so amazing—I love this community." When I started my own informal cross-country survey, people spoke about the landscape, the city lights, the community centre, but mostly they talked about each other—their neighbours, their community. Our sense of home is inextricably linked to the people who live there. My neighbourhood is great because I have great neighbours.

What strikes me as beautiful and inspiring is the way in which people work to create better communities. In every city and town in this country, I meet people, lots of people, who work hard to make their communities better. They organize fundraisers, establish networks for older people, reach out to the most disadvantaged and isolated residents. They help make their children's schools better, they volunteer on hospital boards and, every so often, they create opportunities for kids to play sports and be active.

The evidence of our caring is all around us. When we talk to our child's volunteer soccer coach, when we watch a neighbour connect with the elderly woman next door, when we volunteer at the local community centre's sports night for teens, we are reminded that people care about one another. As we begin to connect with neighbours and create opportunities for kids to play, we see small changes that buoy us. Kids are meeting at the basketball hoop once a week, there are kids in the park down the street, and neighbours are stopping to talk before they unload the groceries.

We might begin to wonder whether we should keep our schedules and our kids' schedules a little more open so that this atmosphere of play and community can grow; after all, it's free, it's easy, and it means we don't have to drive somewhere again. Maybe the small joys that result from these small efforts take a little of the edge off our busy lives.

The more children who play in the streets, the safer our streets become for our children.

One of the real challenges of communities today is that these days so many of us go into our homes after work and stay there. Sometimes we take our children to after-school lessons or to sports practices, but rarely do children move into our streets, parks and public spaces. These are places where people used to convene, where children of all ages interacted, where parents connected with other parents to help watch all of the children. When I grew up, I roamed the neighbourhood with the kids on my street. We had pre-set boundaries we were not allowed to wander past, but within those boundaries we were unsupervised. I say "unsupervised," but that was not really the case. The moms in the neighbourhood were out hanging laundry or working in the garden or peeking out the kitchen windows. If we were late for lunch, my parents had only to call a neighbour and someone would know where we had been last seen. There were always watchful eyes on all of us. When I was ten I hung out with one of the older girls on the street quite a bit one summer, and when she suggested going to the local grocer to do some "shopping," I agreed to go—with a degree of trepidation, as the store was definitely out of bounds for me. Inside the store my "friend" showed me how to steal candy. We hadn't even left the store when my mom's station wagon pulled into the parking lot. A neighbour had called my mom when she saw me walk past her house on the way to the store. Believe me, that was the last time I wandered past those boundaries without explicit permission.

What we have to do is move beyond our fears. The simple fact is, the more children who play in the streets, the safer our streets become for our children, If we are out supervising the young children, we can also allow our older ones to meet together in the schoolyards, the playgrounds and the cul-de-sacs of our community.

Governments create most of the infrastructures of our society, including everything from health-care systems to recreation facilities, but many of these programs rely heavily on volunteers and personal connections. Millions of Canadians volunteer. They volunteer for patients' services in hospitals, they become Big

Brothers and Big Sisters, they escort an elderly lady to church each Sunday, they coach their children's T-ball team. Without so many of us choosing to get involved in life around us, our social services system would simply not work. I have only to look at my own world to see parents reading to schoolchildren, people offering to coach in my son's soccer league, the volunteer who locates my friend's room for me when I arrive at the hospital— all of these experiences are better because individuals give of themselves and their time. In fact, volunteering is so mainstream in our communities that it hardly seems exceptional. But when I think of all these busy people—driving to the hospital to help the elderly, giving up a night of relaxation with their families to coach my child, serving food to the homeless one night a month on top of a full-time work and family schedule—I am inspired by how remarkable this giving of self really is. Older people would not connect with their communities, young mothers would be isolated in their homes and neighbourhood children would not know one another if ordinary Canadians weren't taking action on behalf of others.

We don't need to be neighbourhood superheroes—we just need to make a consistent, small effort to be a part of the changes we want to see.

The secret to having the energy and time to volunteer lies in believing that our actions can be small but their impact can be huge. Volunteering to take your puppy to the hospital once a week to help cheer up patients may not change the world, but it will certainly change the day for those people who need a smile and some company. It is easy for our good intentions to become overwhelmed by the reality of our busyness, but only if we lose sight of the fact that we don't need to be neighbourhood superheroes—we just need to make a consistent, small effort to be a part of the changes we want to see.

Walking a group of neighbourhood children to school, I don't feel like I am having a great impact, but I understand that the social impact is enormous. Can you imagine how significantly we could change the look and feel of our streets if children used the roads to walk to school? With time, there would be more paths, more older people walking, a stronger sense of connection between neighbours. There would be fewer cars, less pollution, safer streets. Kids would be healthier from the exercise they get walking, and they might even develop a lifelong habit of walking to their destinations. All of this from walking a group of kids to school.

There are thousands of people who know intuitively or through their own experiences that children need opportunities to play, that sport and play are an important part of creating a healthy community for our children. They take action that is often simple, like putting up a basketball net in their local schoolyard, like finding a neighbour to coach the kids who show up at the church to play ball. Great or small, such action is always deeply inspiring and the result of visionary thinking.

Erin Hoops began as a basketball club that ran out of a high school gym in Erin, Ontario. A few years ago the fees for use of the gym rose from $1.71 an hour to $100 an hour. Patrick Suessmuth, the director of Erin Hoops, lobbied both the school board and the town to relieve the club of that astronomical price but lost on both fronts. "In the process of fighting to save Erin Hoops," Patrick says, "I realized that this was not only a battle for a basketball club, but a battle to preserve a fundamental value in our community— affordable recreation." Instead of giving up, Patrick found an abandoned elementary school gym to rent and, with local support and his own money, he was able to open a free gym that kids have access to forty hours a week. The new gym's court was too small for a full basketball club, so Patrick turned it into a community centre where kids could also play basketball. The low baskets were just the right height for younger kids to practise their game and for older ones to perfect their dunks. He bought toys at garage sales and had the community donate games, furniture and a refrigerator. "This club continues to grow," he explains, "in part, because we have few rules . . . Our only rules are no hitting and no door slamming. Kids get enough rules at home and at school, where everything has to be so organized."

Walk into the Main Space, the Erin Hoops youth drop-in centre, and you'll see kids playing roller hockey on the gym floor, girls doing handstands in an old classroom, kids shooting hoops, and spirited games being played in every available corner. Patrick runs the centre with an open door, open heart policy: everyone is welcome and everyone is trusted and respected. It is not quite what he envisioned all those years ago when he was advocating to keep affordable basketball in the town of Erin, but from the obvious pride in his voice and the sheer joy that it brings him every day, you know Patrick wouldn't trade any of it. He loves coming to the centre and finding "Thanks, Pat!" scrawled in huge letters across an old chalkboard. He loves when kids burst into tears when it's time to go home. Five hundred kids a month come through the doors of the centre, and Patrick knows and cares deeply for every one of them. He is a full-time volunteer at Erin Hoops, keeping it afloat out of his own pocket and with the occasional government grant.

—

People like Patrick have inspired me to look at my own area of influence, how I can have an effect in my community of Cordova Bay, but also within the larger community of Victoria and, ultimately, the larger community of Canada. I have heard many inspiring stories, but I also know that there are many more people who could be moved into action, with the right idea, the right support and some connection. My strong belief is that there are thousands of people across this country who have a desire to make their communities better. They want leadership on how to create change, and they need proof that change is possible.

Well, the proof is all around us: Laurie Irwin in Sidney, BC, who worked with other parents to create an active playground program in her school; Steve Friesen, who has redefined house-league sports in his school and has 70% of kids participating; Elaine Devlin, who gets kids to eat healthy lunches at school every day by making it worth 10% of their final grade in PE. Change is happening in almost every corner of this country, and when these people start to connect with one another and inspire and support one another, real social change in the area of increased physical activity and healthy living for our kids is inevitable. These people don't think they are inspiring; rather, they are surprised and

even a little embarrassed when I applaud their
efforts. They see themselves as normal people who
are just doing their little bit.

One of the most important ways we can support
such remarkable people and the initiatives they champion is through inspiration, by sharing the stories of
what others nationwide are doing to get kids active
and make their communities better. Seeing what
other people are doing reassures me that I too can
make a difference; their stories help me forge on and
remind me that change is possible.

The Chagnon Foundation is creating enormous
social change in the province of Quebec. It is working
with communities and neighbourhoods to facilitate
environments that enable kids' health and development. The Chagnon Foundation is a *very* large private
foundation. It certainly has the funds to create significant change, but what is most impressive is the intel-
ligence, careful consultation and planning that have
gone into its investments. The foundation asks the
communities it supports to discuss what they feel is
needed to have healthier children; family health,
dropout rates, isolation and poverty have all been
major issues. After four years of testing different
models in these areas, the foundation concluded that
the best choice was to invest early in healthy lifestyles.

The Québec en Forme program, funded jointly

by the Chagnon Foundation and the Quebec government, is guided by a strong belief in the effect of physical activity not only on health, but on social adaptation, on an individual's sense of belonging to a community or a group. The program's goal for children is to create a path of success in the

> When it comes to the neighbourhoods we want to create for our kids, we have to dream big.

school and at home. When surveyed, the mothers of the poorest kids said their concerns were less about food, clothing and shelter than about where they could find a safe park to take their kids to play, or where they could go to swim. "It is always surprising," said Jean-Marc Chouinard, director of QEF, "because you would think they would be concerned about having more food or better shelter, but often we end up concluding that play is at the centre of mankind and is the key relation to our vitality: when you feel and hear your heart going faster, you feel alive." QEF created a partnership with the provincial government and today runs 150 school programs, reaching close to 35,000 kids.

The Foundation is studying ten thousand kids as they move through the program. Chouinard, an Olympian who won an amazing *six* World Cup fencing titles, is in charge of Children and Community

Development. He says, "We are seeing kids who have difficulty at five years old running a few metres and then you see them six months later and they are running across the gym and back—they have so many new abilities. I've seen twelve-year-olds who have never ridden a bicycle before become some of the class hotshots on their bikes." The Chagnon Foundation is playing a significant part in helping the most disadvantaged children in Quebec lead healthier, more positive lives.

When it comes to the neighbourhoods we want to create for our kids, we have to dream big: more opportunity for them to move around freely, a better quality of physical education programs in the schools, a strong network of community play programs available to all children. Many of us remember what we experienced as children—the opportunity to play freely, the programs and clubs built into our schools, the games outside and within our community—and these memories are a powerful compass, pointing us in the direction of what we want for our children. What others are already doing can provide a detailed map.

In creating better communities for our children, belief will be our strongest asset—belief that it is possible, belief that we can work together to achieve it. We can be paralyzed by the sheer immensity of the task of shifting the behaviour of an entire generation of kids. We have to first imagine what we want to create, and what gives us the strength is the evidence that it *is* possible. I tell stories about what ordinary people in this country are doing because these stories inspire me—they make me know that people are creating change and that I can add my voices and actions to the voices and actions of a growing multitude. These stories provide hope that change is within our reach.

> We have to first imagine what we want to create, and what gives us the strength is the evidence that it is possible.

This hope is a crucial part of belief. It is belief that will help us do battle with a city that wants to make it illegal for our kids to play hockey on the street; it is belief that gets me on a plane from Victoria to Ottawa to once again advocate for physical activity as a priority in our health systems. Nobody starts their after-school play program thinking they will inspire others; they do it because it needs to be done, because they see a gap in what is being given to their kids and they want to fill it. But they *do* inspire us, and if we keep telling the stories, if we keep showing ourselves and others what is possible, we begin to build power and momentum.

—

Two years ago, while visiting the Yukon as an inspirational speaker, I learned about the Whole Child Project (WCP) at Whitehorse Elementary School. The project captured my attention because it was doing what so few communities seemed to be able to do: it was using the school as a community centre during after-school hours. One night a week, a school bus makes the rounds through the downtown streets of Whitehorse, picking up kids and parents and bringing them to the school for activities, games and workshops. Anyone and everyone is welcome: grandparents, moms, dads, even people without children of their own.

The WCP began as an initiative in the downtown core of Whitehorse to help parents assist their children in succeeding at school. As in most urban centres, this downtown area is home to many low-income families, homeless people and others struggling with addictions, mental illness and poverty. Whitehorse Elementary is located right in the middle of town, across the street from a Salvation Army soup kitchen, and there are often people taking shelter for the night on the steps of the school. The school is located in an area with the highest crime rate in the Yukon. One might assume that Whitehorse Elementary would be a natural target for vandalism and other related violence because of where it's situated, but it isn't. "According to the RCMP, our school has the lowest incidence of vandalism in the Yukon," says Crystal Pearl-Hodgins, director of the WCP, with obvious pride. "That is at least in part because we have made the school available as a place for kids and parents in the downtown core to feel welcome and safe, a place that they care about. It is a place where people get help and get to know one another; it is a place where people become empowered in their lives."

The first step for the WCP was conducting door-to-door interviews with downtown families. It learned that many families in need either did not know how to access the social services available— whom to call, what forms to fill out, how to get help with employment—or simply did not have the time or energy to do so. The WCP team understood that the issue of children's success in school could not be treated separately from the challenges that these families faced at home, so their approach became more holistic.

Many of the families surveyed did not feel that they could fully participate in the community for reasons that essentially boiled down to two: lack of money and insufficient transportation. The city pool, for example, had recently relocated from the downtown core to the outskirts of town—which was great for all the families who lived in the suburbs and had vehicles, but many downtown families could not make the trip. And if you didn't have a car, you couldn't get there because public transportation shuts down early. Families dealing with poverty, substance abuse and violence already feel isolated from society due to their circumstances, and this kind of city planning tends to isolate them even further.

So Whitehorse Elementary became a focal point for bringing families together. Every Wednesday night, the doors are open to the entire community. And in just four years, the project outgrew the van the Lake Laberge Lions Club had generously donated. It now uses the school bus to provide free transportation, and the school's principal rides along to ensure the safety of any children who come alone.

Open School nights see forty to fifty children, parents and grandparents in classrooms taking cooking classes, learning the craft of stained glass, working through challenges in the Nobody's Perfect parenting workshop, running the halls, playing dodge ball in the gym, chatting and laughing with one another. Open School is premised upon the understanding that if you want to make a difference in families and the community at large, it is not enough to just provide opportunities for children: the *whole* child requires attention, energy and support for the idea of whole families. On Open School nights, kids have the opportunity to be active through co-operative games and dynamic learning environments, and entire families have the opportunity to become healthier and more connected in a welcoming, interactive, educational and supportive environment.

For Barbara Curtis, a former client of the WCP who is now its outreach worker, Open School night was a life raft: "Open School would not allow me to shrivel up. When I say that Open School night got me to shower for the first time that week, that is no word of a lie. When things in my life got really, really bad, this program got me and my kids to a healthy, supportive and fun place to be and it allowed me to be more than just a 'welfare mom.'" There were many weeks when Barbara—at the time an exhausted, unemployed and depressed single parent totally overwhelmed by having to be on time for one more thing—felt that she simply did not have the strength to go, but her kids had become deeply attached to Open School night and would make her. "Sometimes I hated every minute of it because I had to get it together, but I loved when I would get home at night and have a chance to think about the conversations I'd had. After Open School, I was always a little lighter, even in the darkest times."

The WCP is working. The RCMP's National

Youth Strategy, an initiative that invested $50,000 in the project to get it off the ground, sees the positive impact programs like WCP have in communities and in supporting families at risk: reducing crime, reducing crisis and reducing the expense often associated with reactive problem-solving. The WCP's common-sense approach has supported many families in getting the assistance they need; it has allowed young people from all economic situations to enjoy crafts, courses and games together; it has helped young mothers understand the nutritional needs of their babies; it has connected those isolated by poverty and made them part of a vibrant community—one that they not only join, but have a hand in creating. As Barbara recalls,

> When I was in crisis, depression hit me pretty hard, and one of the first things to go was my social life. When people know you are in trouble, you start to avoid them. Open School nights allowed me to be supported and do things that were fun and I was good at— devoting time to doing things for my own peace of mind and my own self was incredible. I could escape into a world where only my imagination existed and could limit me. I got to do things with each of my boys alone.

Special times, just one on one. As a single
mother of three boys, that was one of the hard-
est things to manage. I did crafts with them,
math games, taught them to swim. We were
carving memories every time we came ... The
independence they are all being allowed to
develop and watching them grow is amazing.
They love it, they are happy there, they don't
like to miss it and they bring their friends. It
really is the most meaningful thing I have done
in my whole life, and I love that we are doing it
as a family. And I love that it's my job!

The WCP has helped many families in
Whitehorse. In April 2005, sixty families turned up
for swim night, laughing and celebrating together
with other families, teachers, administrators and volunteers from the RCMP and the community. The
bridges these families are building are smoothing over
years of negative and ineffectual relationships with
their community, its services and each other. The
WCP's success lies in its determination to serve as a
link to the community and services of Whitehorse,
not be a centralized, prescriptive, top-down organization. It is not trying to be the only service in
Whitehorse, as each school or community has its own
unique challenges. Instead, the WCP wants to serve

as an example and as a resource that other schools in Whitehorse can use to launch their own ideas.

The WCP accomplishes so much because it has allowed a great idea to be driven by passionate and compassionate individuals. When asked what advice she would give to anyone who is thinking about getting involved in their own community, Crystal said, "Find out what people need, what they want, where they see the shortfall. Don't just apply your ideas to a situation you may not know that well. Get out and ask, show that you care in concrete ways with your own actions and demonstrate that you are listening to people with a vested interest in making the community a better place to raise your families." Just as Father Mouchet understood, we all need to learn before we can teach—learn about what our families and our communities really need in order to become healthy.

When children play, the world wins!

—Right to Play motto

SPORT FOR PEACE

It is a concept that takes a moment to digest: sport for peace. But what it means for many people is sport brought into refugee camps, sport being encouraged and developed in the most disadvantaged places in the world. But how can sport be as important as food, clothing and shelter?

I had those questions in 1999 when I received a letter from Johann Koss, a four-time Olympic gold medallist in speed skating, on behalf of his organization Right to Play. Johann asked if I would come to Africa to witness how sport was transforming refugee camps in Sudan and Eritrea. I couldn't imagine how sport and play could be nurtured in a refugee camp, and wondered how sport could even be a priority when so many other basic needs were barely being met. But Johann's passion for and belief in his work were irrepressible, and it took him only thirty minutes to convince me that going to Africa would profoundly change my perspective on the importance of play and sport for children. Ten days later, I was on a plane to Khartoum.

We spent a day there sorting out visas, drivers and translators, then headed out to a camp called Laffa, located just inside Sudan's border with Eritrea. We travelled in white UN vehicles under the relentless African sun. Paved roads gave way to dirt roads, which eventually disappeared into an open expanse of desert that our driver navigated expertly. I didn't know how to feel about this landscape of sand-blown hills, ever-present eddies of swirling dust and a sun with absolutely no mercy. It was awe-inspiring, it was beautiful and it was cruel.

After hours of driving, I was able to make out small shadows in the distance that split the sand from the sky. The shadows became tents as we drew nearer—rows upon rows of tents lined up by the hundreds, all the same colour as the dust. I felt excitement that we were finally reaching the camp, but also nervousness about my role during the next few days, and anxiety about what I would feel in face of the poverty and sadness. And then I saw children, hundreds of them, lingering lethargically beside their mothers, kneeling, standing, motionless. Children with absolutely nothing to do. They were not playing, or running, or throwing a ball. But as our SUVs moved in, many jumped up and ran to meet us. Our arrival seemed to generate a lot of excitement—as I descended from the Range Rover, the crowd of children stepped back and pointed at me, repeating "white man" in their language, over and over. I smiled at the children and spoke to them in English, and they giggled and began to come closer. One brave little girl grasped the index finger of my left hand, and a minute later nine more were holding the rest of my fingers. I had an overwhelming desire to pick these little people up and hug them, to give them something, to share some part of me with them.

I began to sing and jump to some skipping songs I remembered from childhood. The children pointed at this big white girl and laughed with glee. Soon I had two hundred children following me around the camp learning ring-around-the-rosy and Marco Polo.

Over the next few days, I participated in setting up play and sport programs in Laffa. The Norwegian coaches who had volunteered to work in this camp would spend the next six months customizing the program to suit the needs of the children. My main role for the ten days I was there was to help document what was happening and to take part in a one-day sports festival. We played with the kids, taught them games and set up a soccer tournament. I showed some little ones how to play hopscotch and they loved it.

On the sports day, all the children in the camp came together to learn and play games like volleyball, soccer and freeze tag. Most of the boys showed up to play, and a lot of girls showed up to stand on the sidelines. I encouraged the girls to join in, but their nervous mothers pulled them away. We were determined to get those girls playing, though, because we could see the interest and excitement in their eyes. Eventually we managed to convince about twenty of them to learn soccer. Many of these girls had never kicked a ball before, and some girls screamed and squealed when the ball came toward them. Shouts of encouragement and good doses of laughter were just the right things to get them kicking the ball. I was startled by how fast they were learning and suggested we move on to playing a game. They said sure, so I divided the girls into teams.

I had an overwhelming desire to pick these little people up and hug them, to give them something, to share some part of me with them.

Sometimes not understanding the rules that govern and divide different cultures and not being familiar with the social and political undercurrents that shape our interactions can be liberating. I had no idea when I put those teams together that I had unwittingly placed Christian and Muslim girls—girls who would *never* voluntarily get together—on the same teams. Although I would never recommend ignorance as a strategy, not understanding what shouldn't be done helped initiate what needed to happen: some seriously fun playtime.

There was no time before the game started to work out religious differences. The Muslim girls simply tied their headscarves at the back of their necks or on the tops of their heads and started to play. The Christian girls got right into the game, too. The mothers fussed a little bit, but because everything was happening so fast, they had no opportunity to shut the game down. I played alongside the girls, none of us really paying attention to the rules except the most important one: get the ball into the opposite net. An hour later, we came off the field sweaty, dusty and exhausted from running and giggling and screaming together the whole time.

Taking a breather, I stood beside a UN worker who had been working in Laffa for three months. She had tears in her eyes as she turned to me and said, "I have never, never seen the children in this camp come together like this. Different religions, boys and girls—it is overwhelming to see."

I went into that camp with little knowledge of the "facts" of these peoples. I didn't know what separated them, I didn't know that girls don't usually participate in sports, but I believed in something that would bring joy and fun to each and every one of them: the power of play. My experiences in Laffa proved to me that every child, no matter his or her circumstance, has a right to be transformed, transported by play.

Today Right to Play works in thirty-six communities throughout Africa, Asia and the Middle East, and emphasizes fairness, equality and inclusion. One of the organization's priorities is empowering the communities it works in by training young local leaders to develop programs that benefit from Right to Play's support and knowledge but aren't completely dependent upon it. Right to Play brings in program coordinators to identify young leaders and then train them to coach and teach children in their community.

I returned to Africa recently, and I was talking to a group of coaches from a camp in Lugufu. They kept joking about "gender balance, gender balance," because it was a message they had heard so often in their RTP training days. The idea of equal gender representation in sport was pretty new for these coaches, and yet they were embracing the challenge of getting more girls playing.

Right to Play encourages participation in the face of the differences that divide people. In Pakistan, Right to Play has been so dedicated to providing opportunities for girls that it helped build a totally fenced-in field so that girls could wear shorts and play together and not worry about being seen or subjected to abusive comments from others. Today, happily, the community has accepted girls playing sports and the fence is no longer needed. Right to Play's core belief is that everyone has a right to play, and the organization is committed to ensuring that opportunity in culturally appropriate contexts. And in areas such as Afghanistan and Africa, long-standing social norms must be challenged to make this a reality because play is not something we inherently value as a right.

The children in such camps deserve a childhood. They need to feel joy; they need to experience hope.

But it is. Play is a right because it is a child's way of getting to know the world. In Tanzania, I visited Lugufu, where more than 170,000 refugees live in five camps. I had always thought of refugee camps as very temporary, but in Lugufu I met an eight-year-old boy who had been born in his camp; in fact, most of the children in the camps had been born there, and the teenagers had spent half their lives inside these "temporary" settlements. The psychological toll of living in these camps can be devastating. The people are not free: they can't cross the designated perimeter of the refugee camp, they can't work, they can't plan for their future. The younger kids can go to school, but there is no secondary school in any of the camps. Their future is completely unknown. They do not know if and when they will be able to go back to Burundi or the Congo. One man asked me if I knew when he would be able to return to the Congo, and I could only shake my head and sympathize with his longing to be home.

The children in such camps deserve a childhood. They need to feel joy; they need to experience hope. Children playing sports have fun: they laugh and have permission to be playful and silly. They learn from their coaches, they follow rules and they build trust for one another, and sports like Ultimate Frisbee, soccer and volleyball become social focal points. The really small children need play as well— they learn that hitting two blocks of wood together makes a sound; they learn that pushing a ball makes it move away from them; they learn that being co-operative makes other kids want to play with them.

Children also deserve positive and high-quality

role models. The coaches who are trained and developed within camps through the Right to Play program have the opportunity to develop leadership skills, take on positions of prestige and be respected within their communities. In Lugufu, I met more than a dozen "master coaches" who had participated in workshops and led enough activities to become qualified trainers of other coaches. I met one master coach named Jasim who had been coaching in Lugufu for three years. He had named his first boy Sean, after a master coach who had worked there and trained him, and his second little boy, who was only six weeks old when I visited, Ryan, after one of Right to Play's program coordinators. Sitting in his tiny home with his wife and two children, Jasim glowed with the pride of being a master coach—his training certificates and a Right to Play poster covered the main wall. Pride. That is the word that kept coming to me as I sat in Jasim's home. Pride in yourself, pride in your family, pride in what you are doing. As a refugee, Jasim has nothing material, no "future" that is clearly defined, yet he has pride and he has hope and he is part of a legacy of well-being that embraces every child and reaches into every corner of his community. He has joined a lineage of well-respected and admired master coaches, people who will be remembered for what they contributed to humanity, not what they took from it.

—

The United Nations Convention on the Rights of the Child came into being because children's basic human rights are being violated on a global scale: they are the victims when states take up violence against one another, they starve when economic policies don't work, they are orphaned when their parents die of starvation or AIDS, and they are even being used to fight adults' wars. Children are being robbed of a quality of life that they deserve—they deserve to know joy, health, well-being and peace. They deserve to know and experience play, and this right is now clearly enshrined in the UN's Convention—which has become the most widely accepted human rights treaty in history, ratified as of the beginning of 2006 by 192 countries.

While I was in Africa, I spoke with Dyonne Burgers, the manager of Right to Play's programs in Tanzania. She had spent the previous two years working in Sierra Leone, where the human rights of children have been brutally violated during a guerrilla war fuelled by the desire to control diamond mines. Children in that country have been ruthlessly targeted and employed as soldiers. They have been kidnapped, drugged and forced to kill members of their own families or face their own deaths. The guerrillas terrorize the countryside, sometimes chopping off the limbs of children and adults as a strategy of intimidation. Personally, I can barely digest the thought of these atrocities; they seem too terrible to be real.

> Kids don't define themselves as sick or dying or traumatized; rather, they live in the moment, and they seize as much fun and joy as possible.

While speaking to Dyonne, I said I didn't think I could ever go to Sierra Leone, that I wasn't sure I could handle the collective pain and horror that has been experienced by the country. She then surprised me by telling me that the two years she spent there were among the most beautiful and rewarding of her life:

> The people I worked with in Sierra Leone had a ferocious determination to get on with their life. The kids had been traumatized—there were kids that you knew were probably never going to be able to emotionally recover from the trauma—but even some of the children who had experienced the worst situations responded very positively to the play and sports programs we helped create. One of our coaches at the camp had been a child soldier, and he is now a great leader and coach for the other children. You think that it would be

tragic and sad, and it is, but what I felt most was hope and determination. These people want to get on with their life; the kids want to play and be kids, and they all deserve help in moving forward.

In my own life, I have often witnessed the amazing resiliency of children. Justin Verdiel, a little boy to whom I grew very close while he was battling cancer and staying at the Ronald McDonald House in Toronto, seemed sick only when he was in pain. For those days and moments, he acted and was sick; for all the other moments, he was just a kid—he wanted to play and be with his friends and tease his parents. While at Ronald McDonald House, any moment he wasn't feeling weak or sick he would run outside to play hockey. Even while I was with him in Sudbury during the last week of his life, he would ask me if he could go outside and ride his horse or play hockey. Kids don't define themselves as sick or dying or traumatized; rather, they live in the moment, and they seize as much fun and joy as possible. It is adults, particularly those of us who are not close to the tragedy or trauma at hand, who define a child by what has happened to him or her. Really, children have a lot to teach us about life and loss.

In addition to introducing sports and play into

places where children have had little opportunity to be playful, Right to Play has created programs that specifically teach health messages through play. Their Live Safe, Play Safe program focuses on HIV/AIDS awareness. In Tanzania, I played some of the games with the children. We learned about how viruses spread by playing a game in which one child, who was the "germ," would touch another child, and then the second child would run around a circle; if he managed to get to the "doctor" and receive a vaccination, he'd be safe. When they were tested a month later for their message retention, the kids not only remembered the games, they remembered the messages.

When Right to Play began its work in camps in both Eritrea and Sudan, there were no sport programs, no fun activities for children, and girls were not allowed to play. The kind of coming together that Right to Play facilitates has created an unexpected activism. The coaches became the ones who encouraged girls to participate and have fun. And although the mothers were reluctant at first, once they saw the joy in their daughters' faces as they played, they made sure the girls could continue. The mothers helped the girls get shorts so they could run faster, and they supported them through a huge cultural shift in their community.

The mothers became very vocal, insisting their daughters have access to the Live Safe, Play Safe program, even in the face of resistance from their men. They advocated fiercely on behalf of their children, stating, "We want to protect our children from AIDS, and we want them to know how to protect themselves." Soon, the mothers began telling Right to Play what they needed most and even assisted in making many of the current programs a reality.

Johann Koss told me one story that was particularly inspiring:

> There was a seventeen-year-old girl in our program in Eritrea. She was incredible; she was a mobilizer, getting other kids involved in our programs, talking to moms about letting their girls play. She really became a huge spokesperson for Right to Play. She had a two-year-old and at one point was badly burned on the arm when an oil lamp spilled. She became depressed because she had trouble doing the sports she had become so committed to, but she managed to pull herself out of that depression. She enrolled herself in high school and set her sights on training for university. She did this because she wanted to create a better life for herself and her child, and she believes

she got the self-confidence because of what she had been able to do through sport. Sport helped her to believe in herself. It has a transforming effect: it builds hope, opens people up to new possibilities and helps them become stronger. In Eritrea, it showed the women and girls what is possible for them and gave them a voice in their communities and families.

When Johann Koss first boarded a plane destined for Africa, most of the seats had been taken out to make room for boxes of sports equipment—thirteen tons to be exact, all donated by Norwegians. One journalist took offence at Johann's bringing sporting goods to Eritrea, claiming that what Africa needed was food, water and medicine. But Eritrean president Isaias Afwerki greeted Johann and his team with open arms, and more than one hundred thousand children lined the streets as Johann made his way to a mostly demolished stadium with shoes and balls for the kids. "Thank you, thank you," the president exclaimed, "for treating us like human beings. Your sport builds hope, and hope is what will heal this country."

It was while in Eritrea that first time that Johann experienced a moment that brought home to him the power of sport to positively influence children's lives.

He was standing on the street when he noticed a small group of boys gathered by a poster showing young militia fighters. They stood in a circle and seemed almost mesmerized by the poster, which encouraged boys to join the army. A second later, the first group in a cycling competition flew by, and the boys all turned their heads and started cheering and running after the bikes. Johann knew then that "the boys needed other kinds of role models besides men with guns to look up to."

War is an unsettling and cruel reality in the lives of far too many of the world's children. Helping children heal is Right to Play's primary emphasis in Sierra Leone, where, through sports programs, child soldiers are reintegrated into their communities. It is hard to put the words "child" and "soldier" in the same phrase; it is impossible to imagine a nine-year-old child being drugged, kidnapped, forced into a life of violent combat and taught to kill other children. The inherent fearlessness of childhood that makes children brave and adventurous and creative in a healthy context is preyed upon by guerrilla leaders, who make "soldiers" out of kids in destabilized regions. If the children are lucky, they survive—only to go home to communities where the people who once loved them are now afraid of them, to communities and families ill-equipped to help these children heal.

"As soldiers, these children looked up to the young men that were their leaders," says Johann. "They were part of a rigid social order where disobedience meant torture or death. No matter how misguided and evil, without this social order, these children's worlds fall apart. As well, by the time they are young adults, they are fully

By playing with others, these damaged children can rediscover what it means to belong.

aware of the consequences and implications of their actions; they are haunted by nightmares, feel intense anger and shame, and many of them just want to die." But when local children and former child soldiers play on soccer teams together, the former soldiers can not only become kids again, but help their community to see them as kids again. By playing with others, these damaged children can rediscover what it means to belong. In the Lugufu camp in Tanzania, where guerrilla leaders have tried to recruit young adolescents as soldiers, none of the kids have joined, primarily because they have something else that engages them, gives them a sense of belonging and provides a sense of possibility—sport and play.

Sport is a context in which these children can find structure and order: rules are established, there are team leaders to look up to and positions to play, and there is a coach to help keep it all together. Sport also provides a place for a community to come together to cheer its kids on and connect with one another. It fosters friendship, co-operation and feelings of goodwill that strengthen the fabric of a culture.

"Sport is a great equalizer; it doesn't matter where you're from or what your skin colour is or what your religious affiliations are, if you can play, people are going to want to play with you."

Right to Play has recently teamed up with an organization called Playing for Peace to bring basketball to Palestinian, Israeli-Arab and Jewish children in the West Bank. In August 2005, these groups ran week-long overnight camps that brought 130 kids from these three backgrounds together. The camps mark the genesis of a year-round program that will set up twin basketball schools in Israeli-Arab and Jewish villages, where the kids will play separately two or three times per week and then meet for a joint activity once or twice a month.

Playing for Peace was founded upon a distinct premise: "Children who learn to play together can learn to live together." It is a belief that executive director and co-founder Brendan Tuohey just calls "common sense." As Brendan explained to me, "My brothers [and co-founders of Playing for Peace] and I grew up in a pretty diverse neighbourhood and we just realized that sport is a great equalizer; it doesn't matter where you're from or what your skin colour is or what your religious affiliations are—if you can play, people are going to want to play with you. When you are playing, none of those things matter; what matters is whether you can make a layup. Someone will pass you the ball if you can do that. Sport universally breaks down barriers—you start giving each other high-fives and you forget that you're not supposed to like somebody. It's not necessarily a new concept, but it's such a simple one."

Simple enough to build an international organization on—what began as three American brothers playing competitive basketball and coaching in Ireland has grown into a program with coaches, camps, courts and kids in three countries. In Northern Ireland, Playing for Peace brings Catholic and Protestant children together to play basketball in school and in competitive clubs. In South Africa, white children are bussed out to the black townships for tournaments and games. On any given day, and between the two places, Playing for Peace has more than one hundred local coaches working with thousands of kids playing basketball.

Brendan has many inspiring stories about the

success of Playing for Peace: "In Northern Ireland, kids who would never have talked to each other, much less played with each other, are meeting on the basketball court. Now we're seeing them on the street saying hello and becoming friends. We were at a tournament once and the local media interviewed two kids from the same team. The boys were asked how they met and they said they met at the basketball club. They were asked if they were the same religion and they didn't know. It turns out one was Catholic, the other Protestant. They looked at each other kind of shocked, and the interviewer asked whether or not it mattered. They both said, 'No!' You could see at first that they were stunned to realize they were different, but then they both just kind of shrugged and said, 'Whatever,' and went back to playing."

Brendan also shared a story about the first time they bussed those white schoolchildren out to a black township to play basketball:

People thought we were crazy, that the townships were too dangerous. But my brother and I had gone out ourselves a year earlier and had done the groundwork, so that helped us establish some trust with the parents. The South African Broadcasting Corporation followed because it was the first time this had happened.

In the video, you see the kids get all quiet and nervous because they've never been to a township. Waiting for them when the bus pulls up is a group of kids from the township school singing songs and clapping. The kids get off the bus and are greeted with friendship flags and handshakes. And then they just start playing with each other! Later, the captain from the black school and the captain from the white school were interviewed. The white kid talked about how nervous he had been before he came and how great the experience was and how he couldn't wait to come back. The black kid also said he was nervous about having the white kids come, but he realized that they [the township children] were just as good, that they were equals. Now this is happening on a weekly basis and the result is that coming together is not such a big deal anymore. Kids are getting used to seeing each other a lot more.

Anyone who has followed the news in Northern Ireland, South Africa and the West Bank understands the magnitude of this simple shift. Children who have been typically antagonistic toward each other are now having to pull together as a team, make passes to, communicate with and support each other.

Children who have been taught by their parents and their communities to fear and despise each other are laughing together, throwing encouraging arms around each other and saying hello on the streets where their parents fought.

When asked how he would respond to anyone who thinks that bringing play and sport to regions destabilized by political, social and cultural tensions or by poverty and sickness should not be a priority, Brendan is adamant: "They're wrong. Playing is a human right. Sport, for kids growing up, is the most basic outlet you have for fun, socializing and learning. A lot of problems happen when kids lack constructive outlets; when we take those outlets away from our kids because of our fear and ignorance, we leave them only negative alternatives for coping. Play is a human right and we've got to support *every* kid playing. It's a great way to educate; it's healthy for kids to be active and learn great life lessons: how to win, how to lose, how to set a goal and reach it, how to work as a team."

Seeing the impact that organizations like Playing for Peace and Right to Play are having in troubled areas of the world, witnessing how children were changed by the experience of playing together, watching girls of different religions play soccer together—all this solidified my belief in the sheer power of sport and play. Sport has a transforming effect for all children, and kids are too often not being allowed to benefit, even in affluent areas in North America. In the cities and towns of our own countries, we have disadvantaged kids, kids who deserve to be given the opportunity to play in a safe and supportive environment. Johann was right when he said my trip to Africa would intensify my belief in the importance of play and sport for children. As it has turned out, my involvement with Right to Play has become a touch-stone for all the work I do concerning physical activity and kids here in Canada. What Right to Play does has inspired me to bring the joys and lessons of sport to as many children as possible in my own country.

"Mommy, sometimes do you have a dream, and then you wake up, and then you find out your dream is real? I do."

KATE, AGE 6

DREAMING INTO ACTION

Silken's Active Kids Movement (SAKM) was born out of the desire to create opportunities for kids to play. It is premised upon the belief that unstructured play, sport and games are an invaluable and non-negotiable part of childhood. It is built around the games most of us used to play, and encourages us to dream up new ones with our kids. Silken's Active Kids Movement refuses to accept the current state of communities and neighbourhoods as an unchange-able reality; instead, it sees the potential for change. That potential is in all of us: parents, teachers, kids, relatives, neighbours. SAKM delivers on the promise that all children, regardless of their economic background, have the right to play games and sports without cost, referees or intense competition. All children have the right to discover the joy of moving their bodies with their friends and parents and neighbours.

In the days and months following that conversation on the plane with Ric Young, I talked with my business manager, Sandra Hamilton, about what I could do. I also paid attention to what other people working in the areas of play and physical activity were doing. Sandra and I discovered that there were hundreds of groups running programs focused on getting kids active. We found countless websites, brochures, facts and interesting ideas, but the information, aside from being overwhelming in sheer quantity, seemed not to be connected very well. For instance, there are great programs out there supporting low-income families who want to put their kids into sports, but nobody at my community centre knows about them. Sometimes connecting people to resources really does require having someone with what Barbara Curtis at the Whole Child Project calls "a Ph.D. in paperwork."

I decided that I wanted to focus my energy on increasing physical activity in Canadian children, and I started to ask, what can I do and where will I be most effective?—the very same questions that many other

Canadians were also starting to ask as our knowledge of the childhood obesity epidemic increased.

On National Child Day, November 20, 2003, the Senate on Parliament Hill in Ottawa was full of hundreds of children. I was talking about the importance of play and the joy to be found in moving our bodies. We pulled out the skipping ropes and many children joined me to skip right there in front of the usually very sedate Senate thrones. It was a happy, joyful and somewhat unusual scene that was picked up by the media and that ran in newspapers across the country.

I immediately became an advocate for physical activity, and I began to hear from champions and organizations all across the country that also cared passionately about this issue and were working to make a difference. Hundreds of conversations later, I was able to answer my own question of what I could do and where I would be most effective.

I had heard from concerned parents looking for guidance; I had listened as community volunteers told me they felt isolated and unsupported, making them prone to burnout. They wanted inspiration, resources and a connection to others so that they could be more effective at taking action and creating change. I also learned that Canada has a wealth of not-for-profit organizations that make a tremendous difference in the health and lives of our kids. Most of these groups are operating on a shoestring budget and lack the necessary resources to adequately promote their excellent programs.

I had no desire to duplicate anyone's effort. What I wanted to do was make it as easy as possible for people to take action. What was needed was a hub of good ideas, resources and a support network for these like-minded incredible community champions.

A year later, with the generous help of Lululemon Athletica and Legacies Now, I launched the Silken Laumann Active Kids Movement, a national charity dedicated to getting more kids active and to promoting the power of play. In direct response to volunteer feedback, we work to provide five key elements essential in moving people into action: Inspiration, Education, Activation, Connection and Celebration.

In 1997, Jane Holmes, a parent I've mentioned before, was horrified to learn that her kids were being fed fast food at their school, Port Williams Elementary in Nova Scotia. Jane was ahead of her time, asking why we were allowing unhealthy food to be fed to our kids on a regular basis in a place where they should be learning about health and good choices. Jane found that many other parents at the school felt the same way. The school agreed to let Jane lead the changes, but first the parents had to guarantee that there would be no loss to the fundraising profits essential to running many of the school's programs. These innovative parents opened a healthy cafeteria in the school, volunteered their time to run it and later added a breakfast program for the children they knew were arriving at school hungry.

For three years this group got local businesses to provide fresh fruit every day at the school, and also had the pop machines replaced with cold milk and water machines. A subsequent $184,000 Health Canada Diabetes Prevention grant allowed for the project to be expanded to eight schools across Nova Scotia, and a project coordinator was hired to take some of the pressure off the pioneering parents. Jane Holmes said no to fast food and took action to create change. Little did she know that in just a few years Nova Scotia would lead the country with an aggressive new food policy that banned all junk food from its schools.

I get so inspired when I hear stories like these— solid proof of what others are doing to get our kids healthy and active, proof that small changes in our families and communities can provide big benefits to our children.

At Silken's Active Kids we are sharing these stories—stories about what your neighbours and community leaders are doing; stories about people who are changing the world. They are not ending world hunger or finding a cure for cancer, but they are making a big difference.

They are parents like running-shop owner Rob Read, who inspires the running club at Victoria's Margaret Jenkins School that has half the children in the school running. Parents like Joanna Fox, who started a school swim club. Or Olympians like Simon Whitfield, who regularly goes into schools to talk to kids about their dreams and the importance of being physically active. At a recreation conference, I was told by an excited Vermilion resident about the Alberta town's program MOVE (Making Our Vermilion Energized), which offers open gym nights for families, swim nights and school health fairs. Ordinary people are already taking up the fight for our kids' quality of life and their health—people and organizations that have sensibly, practically and resourcefully found ways to get kids more active.

These stories help us understand that each of us has a sphere of influence, that every single one of us can do something to provide a healthier, more active life for our kids. At SAKM we celebrate the good that is happening around play and we want to inspire change by talking about it and by providing evidence that it exists abundantly in our communities.

We also want to share ideas. If you are looking

for ideas on how to get your child's school active, you shouldn't have to reinvent the wheel. Parents are busy enough. SAKM wants to help you connect to the resources that already exist, to people who have already done similar things in their own children's schools and to the funders or community partners that can help.

Central to our organization is the Community Action Network (CAN), a support system that makes it easier for people to take a great idea and make it happen. Sudbury CAN, Calgary CAN, Ottawa CAN—it is an empowering acronym. I came up with the name because as a young rower I saw a poster of Olympic gold medal rowers Roger Jackson and George Hungerford on a changeroom wall. Under their beaming faces and radiant gold medals was written "You can too." I would look at that poster every day.

We want to spread that "you can too" mindset. A CAN is a group of people who want to work together in their neighbourhood or community to create opportunities for kids to be active. When people ask, "What can I do to make a difference?" SAKM takes them through the steps of setting up their own community network. We will usually suggest starting in your own backyard. Make time for unstructured play and get outside with your children. Invite the neighbour's kids over, print the recipe cards of games from our website, and offer to supervise your backyard, cul-de-sac or block. Teach the neighbours some great new games to play. Eventually, you may find yourself setting up your own Play in the Park day.

Play in the Park day is my dream—a dream to have one day a week where parents stay after school to play with their children. At my kids' school parent P. J. Naylor and I created Games on the Green, and it is so successful that 75% of the school's children now stay after school every Wednesday to enjoy unstructured play. Play in the Park is something almost anybody can do. Meet with a few neighbours, decide what day one of you can watch over the park, tell everyone that between five o'clock and six-thirty kids are welcome to come and play, and presto—you have Play in the Park. When kids come together in a park, play happens without the grown-ups doing much of anything. One kids says, "Want to play tag?" and suddenly there are a dozen kids running under the swing set, across the green space and over the path.

As you connect with your neighbours, you might start to have ideas that expand upon Play in the Park. Pursue them! A retired pediatric nurse, Sandy Boucher, from Midland, Ontario, has started a group called "Let's Get Physical," which consists of a teacher, local counsellors, health professionals and Olympian Angela Schmidt-Foster. They use their shared expertise and passion to create ways to get kids in their community healthy and active. In our community we are thinking about creating an open gym night at the local school; we are also considering recruiting neighbourhood kids for a regular game of road hockey.

Verlee Hagley, of the Rouleau, Saskatchewan CAN (currently the smallest community in Canada operating an initiative), was one of the first people to contact Silken's Active Kids, and when she heard some of the ideas, she was also one of the first to take action.

First, she pointed out that Play in the Park might not be possible in mid-winter Saskatchewan, but she would work to create a Play in the School community night, similar to the Whole Child Project at Whitehorse Elementary. A committee of teachers, parents and one town administrator armed with some resources from our website very quickly negotiated weekly access to the local school on Wednesday nights.

There would be cooking lessons in the school kitchen, floor hockey and volleyball in the gym. The Roughriders cheerleaders would come in to teach a session or two; there would be yoga, meditation, a photography class and even treasure hunts for the little ones. Verlee secured some money from the TV show *Corner Gas* to fund art and drama programs so there could also be dress-up, dancing and karaoke. She started with the ideas from SAKM and adapted and expanded them for her community.

Do we ever really lose the desire to connect with people, to play together and have fun? Cold Canadian winters can isolate us from one another, but on Wednesday nights in the tiny town of Rouleau, everyone comes out to play.

Keen to influence the activity levels of children in her neighbourhood on Pender Island, BC, Sandra Hamilton decided to try the walking school bus idea: "We and three other families live 3.5 km from the school bus stop. Each day, four cars drove down the same road at the same time, none of us capable of picking up all the children."

Unable to coordinate a daily commitment to walking the children home, the four families agreed to make Thursday the "Walking School Bus Day." The children actually really looked forward to walking home together, and along with beach stops it could often take an hour. The children almost always wanted to continue playing together and would often not arrive home until just before dinner. When they were driven home, they were isolated within their own homes and did not venture out to play together. Now they are getting more exercise and more play-time and they love it. Sandra says:

The Walking School Bus became so much fun that children were asking to get off the bus so they could walk home with us. Yes, children are asking to walk 3.5 kilometres uphill at the end of their school day! They really do have much more energy than we realize. Interestingly, many adults who heard about the Walking School Bus felt it was too much for the children. The children have never voiced such concerns. Perhaps we have grown so sedentary that we have forgotten just what children are capable of.

All of us are working mums, and we quickly realized a quite unexpected bonus of the plan. Previously, all four of us had to finish work at 3:15 in time to meet the 3:30 bus. But the Walking School Bus is a one-hour pleasure once a month, and it allows the three other mums an extra one and a half hours of work, exercise or meal preparation time three Thursdays each month. Exercise and playtime for children that actually creates time for Mum—now that's a good idea.

Part of SAKM has me speaking to communities across the country about the importance of keeping our kids active; about unscheduling their time, limiting access to the television and the isolation of technology; about creating a little bit more connection in our communities. I am also talking to health ministers and sport ministers, to mayors and city councillors, to premiers, to medical schools and doctors, and to whomever else can help move forward the health of our children. Change has to happen at all levels—individuals can do some, organizations some, and governments can play an integral role. I am not the only one speaking—there are dozens and dozens of passionate advocates of physical activity and kids

As you connect with your neighbours, you might start to have ideas that expand upon Play in the Park. Pursue them!

who speak in their own areas of influence. Together we will create a cacophony too loud to ignore.

The message of the joy that play brings our children—what it does to their minds and souls and bodies—needs to be told. We need to hear it; it needs to resonate for us, and we can then become passionate advocates for the quality and quantity of our children's play. So part of our job at SAKM is to tell that tale, through speaking, through magazine articles and media interviews, through this book. I believe there is tremendous value in articulating clearly what most of us know intuitively: physical play is essential to the well-being of our children.

—

In a world that nurtures feeling helpless over feeling empowered, where many believe we can't make a difference, we need to join together to remind each other that we are not alone, that our simple ideas are good ones, that what we do works. SAKM does not tell people what to do or pretend there is only one way to do things; rather, it seeks to provide the space and Feeling overwhelmed breeds apathy, and believing a problem is too big to tackle will eventually result in a problem too big to tackle because everyone will have lost hope. support for people to be creative on behalf of their kids and communities, and to be a light for others.

We cannot afford to merely exist in our communities; we cannot afford the time and energy spent bracing for the worst while we wait for things to get better. We need to take responsibility for everything we see happening in our communities, because they are a reflection of ourselves.

An action that seems small can have an enormous impact. The people I have interviewed for this book share the perspective that what they are doing isn't that great, that there must be better stories than theirs to tell. But as I said before, my heroes are everyday Canadians. These remarkable individuals each began with a dream that evolved into an idea. Then they took the small steps to make it a reality. None of them thought, "Does this count as effective social change?" They just did what their hearts told them to do.

We have come to believe that everything worth doing must be complicated. This belief is so fervently held that we distrust anything that seems simple. During the first meeting of our neighbourhood CAN, we agreed to start a Play in the Park day every Monday night. One mom started talking about waivers and email addresses and emergency contact numbers. I couldn't see why we couldn't just put up a few posters and hope people showed up. I don't mean to make light of people's concerns, but no wonder we turn back before we even get started! I can tell you that if I had to get a lawyer to write me a waiver and had to set up an email address list and distribution process for all the interested people in my neighbourhood, on top of keeping track of everybody's emergency contact numbers, CAN would still be an idea collecting dust in my head. I never would have gotten out the door. Feeling overwhelmed breeds apathy, and believing a problem is too big to tackle will eventually result in a problem too big to tackle because everyone will have lost hope. Communities can change; families can be transformed; bad habits can be broken and replaced with healthier ones. Change is evident all around us—change is the key to our survival.

SAKM is a place to tell the inspirational stories of change. Some people choose to take action in ways that effect change more dramatically or more quickly; others will hit upon the right idea at the right time and the benefit of this synergy will be slower, smaller, but just as lasting. As we find the courage and energy to effect change in our neighbourhoods and communities and begin to share our stories, we notice we are not alone. Buoyed by the success of others and intrigued by their challenges, we will always be inspired to keep going.

"Mommy, when we go really, really fast, I think we are flying. Do you think this is how it feels to be a bird, Mommy?"

WILLIAM, AGE 8

BOYS ON BIKES

Trotting down the street behind my enthusiastic five-year-old as she rode her bike, I wondered how many kids were going to show up for our second neighbourhood Play in the Park day. Twelve kids had shown up the week before, a solid start to establishing regular neighbourhood playtimes. At the end of the narrow street, I saw two boys on bikes, hastily rounding the bend. I hoped that meant they were going to the park to play. Within seconds, six more boys on bikes whizzed by and made the same turn. My heart began to beat a little faster—anticipation? Excitement? I don't know, but in that instant the world seemed exactly as it should be: boys on bikes cruising the neighbourhood. My anxiety about facing an empty park that night began to dissipate. "Where are you going?" I shouted after them. "To the park to play capture-the-flag!" one shouted back. I could have wept with joy, and even felt tears prickling my eyes. Instead, I picked up the pace, closing the gap between my daughter and me.

In that instant the world seemed exactly as it should be: boys on bikes cruising the neighbourhood.

Twenty-one kids came to play in the park tonight. They taught us a game called "grounders," a game I had never played before. One person has to walk blindfolded around the play apparatus, trying to catch one of the kids clambering all over it. When the person who is It yells "grounders," the last one to climb back on the apparatus automatically becomes It. One of the girls brought her skipping rope, and a few of the adults tried to teach the little ones to skip. None of the older girls knew any skipping songs, so some moms pitched in and tried hard to remember how those songs went. My mission for next time is to track down a few of those songs so we can all learn them together.

When I asked who wanted to play capture-the-flag, ten children shouted out, "I do!" "Me!" "Me too!"

We dragged some reluctant parents onto the field with a loud cry of "Let's play capture-the-flag," and the game began to take shape. Rules were reviewed, teams created, borders drawn. Suddenly, there were people running in all different directions, adults and kids working together to devise strategies to capture that flag. Fourteen-year-old James helped seven-year-old Nicholas free their teammates; kids chased their parents, who had ended up on the opposing team. Everyone laughed out loud at some point. Kids screamed and careered around. Neighbours exchanged high-fives and good-naturedly teased each other. Every ten minutes or so, someone would do the victory dance across a border, shouting, "We won! We won! We won!"

I feel hopeful, optimistic and buoyed by the evidence of passion and change I see all around me.

This has been my dream, exactly what I experienced tonight: kids running, neighbours talking and laughing, all of us coming together to play. The idea of a neighbourhood Play in the Park day is so simple, and making it happen was even simpler—all it required was a few hours of calling neighbours and putting up flyers. No waivers, no insurance, no commuting, no cost. I thought about my initial hesitation to put my neck out there to try to make this happen, wishing someone else would do it for me so I could just show up, but I'm glad I didn't put it off. The success of this evening is yet another example of small changes having a big significance.

This is the delight that Verlee Hagley must have experienced when she was organizing a community night in her town. SAKM got an email from her shortly after she got started that began with "Yahoo! The town has voted to open the gym!" Perhaps Father Mouchet felt his own version of this joy on cold, snowy days as he watched his young skiers glide along the trails of Old Crow. It is what Jane Holmes must have felt when she witnessed a room full of children eating fruit instead of fries during lunch hour. And that is how I feel as I write these final pages of this book, after all the bad news, after all the moments I have felt red with rage at what is *not* happening in many schools, at parents who simply can't accept where their responsibility lies, at those cynics who say that's just the way it is. Even after all the facts and statistics screaming to us that our children are in trouble, I feel hopeful, optimistic and buoyed by the evidence of passion and change I see all around me.

Any time I am faced with yet another "realist" who tells me that the world has changed, I think of all the champions I have met through SAKM and in the process of writing this book. When someone suggests a problem is too big for one person or asks me how I am going to fight a losing battle against computers, video games and the veritable army of marketers competing for my children's attention and desires, I think of them, of their actions and successes. The thing is, I don't have the answer. I can't really think too much about the marketers or the makers of video games or TV shows. My coach Mike Spracklen's words come back to me: "Thinking about the boat beside you doesn't make your boat go any faster." So I'm choosing to focus on "my boat"—my area of influence, what *I* can do with my time, my knowledge, my talents, to make things better.

The headlines about our children make us pay attention; the danger is that they can overwhelm us. When the shock of the information wears off, we are devastated by how unfit North American children really are. We feel the burden of collective guilt, of our responsibility. To lessen the impact, we tell ourselves that the world has changed, that kids are different now, that we are powerless and small against the social forces that are making our children unhappy and unwell. But we must take this general outlook and apply it specifically to our *own* kids, those babies we hold in our arms in wonder, those toddlers we buckle into sturdy car seats for the trip across town, those five-year-olds to whom we shout "STOP!" in sharp and terrified voices as cars whiz by. We go through extraordinary effort and worry and stress to keep our children safe.

But somehow, we are *not* keeping our children safe. They are dying of heart disease and diabetes; they are being prescribed antidepressants far more often than they were ten years ago. Their little bodies are not accruing healthy bone to the levels that will make them strong adults. We must see that this is a crisis for our children, that this is about so much more than a few kids who need to lose weight. This crisis is about a generation of children who will not experience their potential, physically, mentally and spiritually. And it is a problem that will not solve itself. If we continue to live in families and communities as we have been, the problem will continue to gain momentum.

We can shift that momentum in a positive direction. We *can* create a positive momentum around the health of our kids. Twenty years ago, women routinely smoked and drank during pregnancy—then we learned it was hurting our babies, and took action. Fifteen years ago, we learned that buckling our children into seatbelts dramatically improved their chances of surviving a vehicle accident, and we've been lugging car seats to daycare and

Grandma's house ever since. Only a few years ago we concluded that breastfeeding should be the first choice for mothers whenever possible, and breastfeeding has risen from 15% to 75%. We have shown we are capable of making real and lasting changes in our behaviour. Today we know that our kids need more physical activity, that they need healthy and active school environments and that they need the opportunity to play outside. We need to be so passionate about the health of our kids that we would defeat any government that wasn't taking action; we would fight any school board that didn't support a healthy, active school environment; we would fight anyone who tells us that street hockey is illegal or that we need a permit to play pick-up soccer in the park.

Our first and most important job is to keep our kids safe and healthy.

We are the primary caregivers for our children. It is all of us as parents who need to commit to knowing what is happening in our schools in terms of physical activity and food policies. We have to stop shrugging our shoulders about how kids have hot dog and pizza day every week and find our voices to protest. Our kids cannot be expected to understand the long-term consequences of bad eating and poor lifestyle choices; it is our responsibility to lead the charge for them until they are able to make their own informed decisions.

Our first and most important job is to keep our kids safe and healthy. Sometimes prioritizing health means we have to fight against ridiculous rules that don't allow kids to run in the playground because they might get hurt, or to play hockey on the street because cars will have to slow down.

Now, I have to warn you, speaking up may get you labelled as a fanatic, or maybe even a crackpot, but for the sake of our children's health, we have to make ourselves heard. Case in point: Last week I was approached by a member of our school's safety committee about an unstructured play area that the primary-grade students use during recess. There were concerns that the area was "unsafe" because the kids climb on the rocks and there is concrete at the base of the play area. I said, probably a little too zealously, when asked what I thought, "Okay, here's what I think. Why don't we just bubble-wrap our kids and then send them outside to play? In fact, why let them go outside at all, because something might happen! Instead, let's protect them and keep them inside, or in such an artificial, unstimulating environment that even a kid couldn't have fun. Yes, let's protect them while they shrivel up from inactivity, allow their imaginations to wilt through lack of proper nourishment, their bodies lose that vigour and spring that most adults would do anything to get back!" As the woman carefully backed away, I realized that perhaps I sounded a little fanatical, but I am really tired of hearing "safety" driving many wellness imperatives right off the priority list. Our unstructured play area is a dream for the students. They get to climb and be in a natural environment, and the teachers love it and know its value. Yes, safety should be a consern, but liability and insurance should not be the first priority for a *play*ground.

Will we take up the fight for the joy factor in our children's lives? Our children are not mini-adults—childhood is unique and imaginative and wonderful. I want to hear a lot more noise coming from the gyms and playgrounds and classrooms of our schools. These squeals and shouts and the rambunctious laughter tell me our kids are playing and moving and being joyful. We have to find the energy and the commitment and the passion to be active participants in the health of our children. We love our children, and our deepest wish is for their happiness.

Before any of that negative and defeatist chit-chat gets in our heads, let's remember it's easy—it's child's play. It is about getting our kids playing again. Playing is what children naturally want to do; it is what a child's body is designed to do. If you set up the right environment for kids, they will play—they will follow their hearts, because what makes them healthy is what they love to do. I believe in Malcolm Gladwell's theory of the tipping point: that little things can make a big difference. If enough people are helping kids get active, if enough kids start playing on our streets and in our parks, if enough people are willing to be involved in positive change and if the resources for how to get started are easy to access, then a critical mass of energy will be created and together we will turn this terrible trend of unhealthy children and unsafe neighbourhoods around.

How do our children get their downtime? When in the day do they have time to decompress, to open their arms and run with joy, to lie in the grass and giggle?

My yoga teacher has instructed me many times that "in order to do, you must first *undo*." For me, walking, doing yoga and being outside allow me the time to discover who I am beyond what I do and what I am to others. Without taking the time to walk and stretch and play, the quality of my life would be substantially reduced. These experiences bring me joy and help me connect with the spirit that guides me. But how do our children get their downtime? When in the day do they have time to decompress, to open their arms and run with joy, to lie in the grass and giggle? How will they release their stress from school, from the big job of learning about the world for the very first time? If this time is important to adults, it is essential to our children—our children whose lives are increasingly overloaded. They need this time to figure out who they are, to connect with other kids in a natural, spontaneous way, to learn how to entertain themselves when there is no schedule or program. These are lessons that will help them live full and rich lives, lives that are balanced between hard work, peacefulness and joy.

In my life I have learned that to have the time, you have to *make* the time. I need to schedule my walks in my calendar. I need to remind myself that walking around the block with my dog and kids is part of being healthy and well. I protect my children's playtime. I resist the notion that my children need to study three hours after school—the school already gets them for seven hours, and my children need time to play and relax. I will not allow my weekends to be consumed by early-morning dance classes, birthday parties or baseball. The weekends are family time. Yes, sports and activities can happen, but I refuse to allow them to dominate the pace and rhythm of the weekend and, ultimately, of our family. If my children are anything like their parents, a time will come where they will be motivated to pursue something with passion, and when it comes we will be driving all over and doing homework until late and keeping dinner warm in the oven. This time will come soon enough, but until it does I want to keep my children searching for chestnuts and playing road hockey with their friends and helping lead our neighbourhood Play in the Park.

I have a vision for my family, but also for our communities. This is my vision:

I see a million more children in parks all across the country. Little ones are digging in the sand and streaking gleefully down the slides; older ones are playing dodge ball and starting a game of tag. I hear laughter, and shouts of "Pass me the ball" and "My turn, my turn." I hear the belly laugh of a child who has seen something funny and just can't stop laughing. These sounds warm me most of all, the shouts and shrieks and guffaws that capture the beauty of playing.

Teenagers are in my vision too—they have found a paved area to play in and have started a pickup game of basketball or are teaching the little ones their playground savvy. And in my vision, children are riding their bikes. They are exploring the neighbourhood with their friends; they are meeting at one another's homes and heading over to the high school to do tricks in the parking lot. And the streets don't seem so dangerous anymore. So many kids are riding their bikes or are out playing that drivers have become more aware. I see that the city has put up a new sign: "Slow down, children playing."

I see adults too. Not one adult for every child, but two adults taking six kids for a long bike ride along the waterfront trail in Toronto; I see another, larger group, a parent and two teachers with a dozen kids, and they are climbing the mountain-bike trails of Courtenay, BC. Best of all, I see parents peeking out their living-room windows, noting who is playing in the driveway, knowing every child by name. I see a mom or a dad coming out of the house to walk their little visitors home; I see them calling out greetings and sharing laughter with their neighbours as they tell stories about what their kids got up to in the backyard.

In the communities I envision, parents are rediscovering the small joys of parenting. They are surprised by how good it feels to be outside in the yard throwing a baseball with their children. They take their dusty ten-speeds out of the garage and join the kids for a lap around the neighbourhood. In this picture I see a dad on inline skates on his way to pick up his daughter and then blading home together. These families are spending less time driving their children around and more time playing together. They are reconnecting with their tweens over games of one-on-one basketball and by walking the neighbourhood together each evening.

This vision is not a fantasy. I have simply taken little moments of what is already happening and expanded them to include every family in every community across Canada. There are parents who believe that there is a different way to be in our families and schools and communities. And as they take action, they are beginning to see and hear and feel real change.

This vision is in motion on our monthly CAN conference call. Stephen Nason heard about Play in the Park and is now going to try Play in the Park and Play on the Ice Rink at the Dovercourt Recreation Centre in Ottawa. Stephen listened to our vision and then personalized it—tweaked it to meet the needs and opportunities in his community. In Peterborough, Ontario, Play in the Park is happening in many schoolyards and playgrounds. In Nanaimo, BC, Gillian Goerzen has created a Play in the Park and is looking to partner with the local RCMP.

Many of these people I know personally, others I have never met, but all of their stories are inspiring. These people make me believe change is not only possible, it is happening. To them, change is not a theoretical idea: it is something they are doing every day. Some of the actions they have taken are large-scale and extraordinary; others are simple and require only a little energy—but they are all an important part of creating change in our communities and our society.

At Silken's Active Kids Movement, what we are doing is working. And what we are asking people to do is simple: find one way you can get kids more active in your community. One night a week you must give yourself permission to live more simply, to play as a family, to connect as a community.

Action is required—to turn off your children's television, to get the computers out of their bedrooms, to take yourself outside and pick up a baseball glove. Action is required to call a neighbour and ask if she wants to meet in the park or stay behind at the school playing field so the kids can play soccer. Action is required to speak to the school and voice your desire to have more physical education, better physical education and more outdoor time in the school day.

Change is happening, and as I write this book, it seems to be gaining incredible momentum: Nova Scotia has banned pop machines from its schools; Alberta and Ontario have mandated thirty minutes of daily physical activity in their schools; PEI is putting physical education specialists into every school. I feel deeply grateful to those of you making changes in your area of influence—you inspire me and help me believe that in only a few years this terrible problem will be a problem of the past.

I know that you will have doubts, as I do—times when your efforts don't feel like they are working, when it seems as if the changes you are making in your family are going against the tide. I encourage you to find one another, to call our help line for support, to talk to a like-minded individual or the person in your community who seems to be leading the charge for healthy kids. Each effort we make in getting our families, our schools, our communities active and healthy does contribute something. There is a warm, knowlegeable community of people out there who have made healthy, active kids their absolute passion and priority in life, and my experience is they are ready and willing to help you.

Action is required—to turn off your children's television, to get the computers out of their bedrooms, to take yourself outside and pick up a baseball glove.

I have always found it helpful to think of a big change in tiny pieces. Starting this book, for example, meant I had to begin writing one thought, one page at a time. The idea of an entire book was overwhelming at the start—and sometimes in the middle or at the end!—but I knew these words would turn into pages, and pages would become a chapter and the chapters would become the book. To make it easier on myself, for the first three months I referred to my book as a "booklet."

It can take a little time to see the evidence. When I was back in training after my accident, I spent every waking second in physio, or rowing or strengthening my damaged leg. For weeks I had little evidence that I was getting better, and I had no guarantee of getting to the starting gates in Barcelona. I had to

What lies between where we are today and where we want to go is belief—belief that we can, belief that we will, belief that it is possible for us to see our dreams become reality.

believe—to believe that all my effort, all the work of my team of physiotherapists and doctors, friends and family, that all of it would add up to something—that it would be enough to get me into the final of the 1992 Olympic Games.

We are all going to work to get our communities healthy, to give our children the opportunity and the encouragement they need to lead active lives. And we are going to do this one little step at a time. We are investing in the future, and we will not always be able to see our progress. But that's okay. We invest, we make changes, we put boundaries on our children's television and video-game time, and we believe—we *believe*—that all of these actions will add up to change. That they will take us closer to the dream we have for the future.

What lies between where we are today and where we want to go is belief—belief that we can, belief that we will, belief that it is possible for us to see our dreams become reality. Sometimes that belief feels like a tiny thread holding our lives together; sometimes it feels like a warm blanket covering and protecting every part of us. I experience belief as being held: that no matter what the struggle I am currently facing, no matter what evidence I am faced with, those arms will not put me down.

I have a bronze medal from the 1992 Olympic Games. Every couple of weeks little people run their hands over it as I go into into schools and community centres across this country to talk to kids. I see their wonder and am reminded that dreams come true, that things we imagine in our heads, *can* be willed into existence. The medal is real, but there is still something about it that remains a little magical. I can't explain how I won a bronze medal ten weeks after that devastating accident. The more time that passes, the more magical and unexplainable it becomes. All I know is that I kept dreaming and believing and trusting. I led—not a company or a country, but the only thing I could lead: myself.

I believe every one of us has one of these medals. Tucked away in a corner cupboard, hidden in an overstuffed drawer or dusty corner of our mind—something that represents us at our very best. Dreaming, believing and leading. Maybe it is a certificate from our university graduation, the first dollar we ever earned, a plan for our dream house, the memory of dancing on the patio with our three-year-old in our arms. We need to find it, dust it off and give it a loving polish. We need to reconnect with that very best part of ourselves and bring that part to our families, our schools and our communities. Our kids need us to be at our very best, so that we can make their world better. It is up to us to lead the way.

GAMES YOU CAN PLAY

TAGGING GAMES

Capture-the-Flag

Capture-the-flag is played in a large field with some hiding spots and obstacles—trees, bushes, parked cars—by two equal teams of at least five players each. The field is divided in half, one area for each team, and a jail is marked at the back of each side. Each team is given five minutes to choose a spot and plant its flag in its own territory. In the most common version of the game, the flag is visible to the opposing team; for an extra twist, it can be hidden. The game is won when one team captures the enemy flag and brings it into its own territory.

1. Once the flags are planted, they cannot be moved except by a member of the enemy team.

2. Players are considered to be in enemy territory if either foot touches that territory.

3. Players captured (tagged) by an enemy player in enemy territory are taken directly to jail.

4. Prisoners can be freed from jail if a free teammate sneaks in or makes a run for it and tags them. Only one prisoner can be rescued at a time by a single player. The two teammates then have free passage back to their territory (but must proceed directly and rapidly).

5. Players may guard their flag but may not go within five metres (about fifteen feet) of it unless an enemy player does first. Then they may follow.

6. If a player is captured in enemy territory with the enemy flag, the flag is planted at the spot of the capture and the player is taken to jail.

7. If the game has not been won within a predetermined period of time (half an hour, perhaps), the team with the most prisoners is declared the winner.

Traditional Tag

Traditional tag is best played in an area with a boundary, like a yard, grassy field or gym, with at least four players. Choose one player to be It—or, if you are a big group, choose more than one person to be It. The person who is It chases the other players, trying to "tag" them—to touch them lightly, anywhere on the body (usually on the arm, leg or back).

1. If a runner gets tagged, roles reverse: It becomes the runner and the runner becomes It.

2. Players may choose to abide by a "no tag-backs" rule. When this rule is in effect, a tagged player cannot immediately reach out to "tag back" the player who just made him or her It.

3. The game is over after a predetermined amount of time, or when everyone is too tired to run anymore.

   In a common variation of traditional tag, It's goal is to tag everyone out, not just one person. As they are tagged, players go to a jail on the sidelines. When everyone is out, the first person tagged becomes It for the next round. This variation is best played with more than one person chosen to be It.

Blind Man's Bluff

Blind man's bluff is a tag game in which the player who is It is blindfolded. This game must be played on a smooth, soft surface—grass is best—and in a relatively small area. The players dart around the "blind man," hooting and clapping as he or she tries to tag them. The first one tagged becomes the new blind man.

Elbow Tag

Elbow tag (sometimes called partner tag) is a variation of traditional tag for which players pair up. This game works well for a big group; a minimum of eight players is required. One player is chosen to be It and another is chosen to be the first runner (in big groups, more than one It and runner may be chosen). All the remaining players pair off and link elbows. The pairs space themselves evenly over the playing area. When the game begins, It chases the runner, attempting to tag him or her.

1. If the runner gets tagged, roles reverse: It becomes the runner and the runner becomes It.
2. To avoid being tagged, the runner can latch onto a pair of players, linking elbows with someone. The other half of the pair must immediately detach— and he or she becomes the new runner.
3. The game ends after a predetermined amount of time, or when everyone is too tired to run anymore.

Amoeba Tag

Amoeba tag should be played with at least eight players.

One player is chosen to be It. When the game begins, It chases the other players, attempting to tag them.

1. As players get tagged, they join with It—all holding hands or each other's clothing to form an "amoeba."

2. Any member of the amoeba can tag a player.

   Eventually, almost everyone is attached together in one huge blob, chasing the last few players around the field.

Turtle Tag

Turtle tag is very similar to traditional tag except that in this game, players can avoid being tagged by lying down on the ground on their backs with their arms and legs in the air, like a turtle on its back. One player is chosen to be It. When the game begins, he or she chases the other players, attempting to tag them.

1. Players are safe as long as their legs, feet, arms and hands are not touching the ground.

2. Players must get up again as soon as It is more than a metre and a half (five feet) away from them.

Freeze Tag

There are two versions of freeze tag.

Freeze Tag I

This game proceeds like traditional tag except that

players may freeze into statues to avoid being tagged. Players run around the field chased by It. To be safe, they must stay completely still when It is near them; if they move, It can tag them "out."

Freeze Tag II

This game proceeds like traditional tag except that when players get tagged, they freeze into statues. There are several variations of freeze tag II. In one version, players "unfreeze" after counting to twenty; in another, called TV tag, they unfreeze when a free player tags them and yells the name of a TV show (each show can be used only once per game); in a third version, frozen players can be brought back to life by a free player crawling between their legs (frozen players stand with legs apart and arms out to the sides). In all of these versions of freeze tag II, the game ends when everyone is frozen, or when a pre-determined amount of time has passed. The first person tagged is It next round.

HIDING GAMES

Hide and Seek

Hide and seek is played with at least four players in a big indoor or outdoor area with lots of hiding places. There is no maximum number of players.

Someone is chosen to be It. A central spot—maybe a tree, a gatepost, a kitchen chair or a sidewalk square—is designated home base. To begin the game, It covers his or her eyes and counts to one hundred at home base while all the other players hide. When It reaches one hundred, he or she yells, "Ready or not, here I come!" then starts looking for the hiding players. It's goal is to find and "count out" all the hiding players. The players' goal is to evade It and get "home free."

1. Players must choose a single hiding place and stay hidden there until they get caught or make a run for home base.

2. It counts players "out" by seeing them in their hiding spots then rushing back to touch home base and calling out their names and where they are hiding—for example, "One, two, three on Jason, hiding behind the car!" The player is then out—eliminated from the game.

3. Hiding players may rush home base at any time. If a player touches home base and yells, "Home free!" before It can count him or her out, the player is "safe."

4. Players who are safe or out must remain on the sidelines of the game until the next round. They may not assist It or other players.

5. The game ends when all the players are either out

or safe, or when the game has gone over a predetermined amount of time. To end the game, It yells,
"Alley, alley, oxen free!" or "Ollie, Ollie, in come
free!" All players still hiding return to home base.
6. The first player counted out will be It in the next
game.

Kick-the-Can

Kick-the-can is best played outside in a big, semi-
open area with lots of hiding places. A minimum of
four players is required (the more players, the better).
To begin, designate as the jail a porch, a patch of sidewalk or any specific area big enough to hold several
players. Choose someone to be It. Next, put a handful
of pebbles into a big can (apple juice cans are perfect)
and stand the can right side up on the ground anywhere. Someone kicks the can to start the game. As
the can tumbles over, the players scatter to hide and It
covers his or her eyes and counts to one hundred.
Then It yells, "Freeze," places the can standing right
side up in the jail and goes out to find the hiding
players.
1. If It spies a player, It runs back to the jail, grabs the
can and calls them "out"—for example, "I see Jolie
behind the rose bush!" The player goes to jail.
2. Prisoners can be freed from jail if a free player
comes out of hiding and rushes in and kicks over

the can before It can run back and call the can-kicker out. Once freed, all the prisoners run out and hide, and It picks up the can, counts to one hundred and starts searching for the fugitives all over again.

3. Unlike in hide and seek, players do not have to choose a single hiding spot. They may move around to evade It or to free prisoners.

4. The game ends when It has all the players in jail or a predetermined amount of time has elapsed. To end the game, It calls out, "Alley, alley, oxen free!" or "Ollie, Ollie, in come free!" All the players still hiding return to the jail area.

Sardines

Sardines is hide and seek in reverse. The game can be played indoors or outdoors and works well in the dark. A minimum of four players is required (the more players, the better). To begin the game, all the players close their eyes and count to one hundred, except the player chosen to be It, who hides. When the players reach one hundred, they yell, "Ready or not, here we come," then split up to search for the person who is It.

1. When a player discovers It's hiding place, he or she must quietly hide there too. One by one, the players find the hiding place and join It there, until

everyone is squashed in together like sardines in a can.

2. The last person still left looking is It in the next round.

BALL GAMES

These games are variations on baseball, with different kinds of balls and bats. Although they are played, broadly, by baseball rules, the games may be adapted to the circumstances. Most adaptations are geared toward small spaces and small teams.

1. Imaginary base-runners, called "ghost runners," may be used when teams are too small to have enough base-runners. When a batter makes a hit, a ghost runner may be placed on first base. The ghost runner advances with hits; if the next batter hits a single, the ghost runner is moved to second base (a second ghost runner is put on first). Ghost runners advance only when "forced" ahead; they stay one base ahead of the runner behind them.

2. The playing field may be irregularly shaped, as long as all players agree on the boundaries and on the locations of foul lines and bases.

3. Any number of bases may be used. A common variation used in small spaces is a triangular field with three bases: first, second and home.

4. In games using a very soft ball, the ball may be tossed at an advancing player to tag him out.

For games with pitchers (soccer baseball, slap ball), at least three players are needed. For punch ball, two can play using ghost runners.

Punch Ball

Punch ball is played with a semi-spongy rubber ball (the blue, red and white kind works best). The hitter's fist is the bat. Players "punch" the ball—they hit the ball with the palm side of their fist, usually in an underhand swinging motion. There is no pitcher. Players "at bat" may use one of several techniques for hitting the ball: they can drop the ball down in front of them and hit it after a bounce; they can toss the ball above their heads and hit it overhand; younger players can hold the ball in one hand and hit it with the other. There is no wrong way to hit the ball, as long as it comes off your fist.

Soccer Baseball

In this game, the pitcher rolls a soccer ball underhand to the player at bat, who kicks it to make a hit.

Slap Ball

In slap ball, the pitcher throws the ball (a semi-spongy rubber ball works best) to the hitter, with a bounce. The hitter slaps it down with the palm of his or her hand to make a hit; the ball must bounce in the infield. Slap ball is suited to limited space.

These are just three of the numerous variations of baseball suitable for the street or the backyard. They can be played with almost any equipment: a badminton racquet and bird, or a beach ball—whatever can be found around the house.

OTHER GROUP GAMES

Red Light, Green Light

Red light, green light is best played with at least four players—three to run and one to be the "Stoplight"—in a big open space. There is no maximum number of players. The game begins with the players lined up along one end of the field, facing the Stoplight, who stands at the other end with his or her back turned to the others. The goal of the game is to be the first player to reach the far end—to reach the Stoplight—without getting caught "running a red light." The player who reaches the end of the field first is the Stoplight for the next round.

1. When the Stoplight yells, "Green light!" the players may run forward. During a green light, the Stoplight must not look at the players.
2. When the Stoplight yells. "Red light!" he or she

turns around quickly to look at the runners. Runners must stop moving immediately. They may fall to the ground or assume any position as long as they are absolutely stationary when the Stoplight turns. Any player who is caught still moving is sent back to the starting line.

3. The length of time between green lights and red lights is decided by the Stoplight, who tries catch the running players off guard with a red light in order to send them back.

HOPSCOTCH

Hopscotch is played on a level surface on which lines can be drawn with chalk or masking tape (the sidewalk, an asphalt driveway, a schoolyard, a basement or playroom) and requires at least two players. A typical hopscotch court alternates between single and doubled numbered squares. The squares should be big enough for players' feet. Players may intersperse the numbered squares with squares marked "safe" or "rest." The court may have as many squares as the players decide, but always begins at "1" and ends with a square marked "home." Each player needs a marker to throw (a coin, a bottle cap, a beanbag, a small rock). The goal of the game is to be the first player to successfully hop the court once for every numbered square. To begin the game, the first player throws a marker into square number one.

1. If the marker touches the border of the square or bounces out, the player forfeits a turn. If the marker falls within the square, the player hops down the entire court starting at the first square.

2. Side-by-side squares may be hopped together, one foot in each square. Single squares must be hopped on one foot. When the player reaches the end, he or she turns around and hops back, picking up the marker without falling over or otherwise touching the ground. Players may not hop in the square with the marker still in it.

3. If, at any time while hopping, a player puts a foot down on a line, misses a square, hops in the square with the marker, puts two feet down in a square or stumbles, he or she forfeits the turn, and the next player begins. "Safe," "rest" and "home" squares are neutral and can be hopped through in any manner without penalty.

4. If the player successfully hops the court with the marker in square one, he or she continues the turn by throwing the marker into square two and attempting to hop the court again.

5. Players begin their next turn by throwing their marker into the square they forfeited their previous turn.

SKIPPING

Traditional Skipping

Generally, three players are required for traditional skipping: one to skip and two to turn the long skipping rope (in a pinch, one end of the rope can be tied to a fencepost). The goal of all skipping games is to complete the song and all the actions (jumping in and out, touching the ground, fancy kicks, answering questions, skipping very fast, etc.) without tripping, stumbling or otherwise getting tangled up in the skipping rope. The rope turners lead the singing.

For an added challenge, advanced players can jump two skipping ropes at the same time—a variation called double dutch. For double dutch, the rope turners turn two ropes overhead at the same time, one after another, creating a syncopated rhythm. Skippers have to jump double-time.

Single-Skipper Games

Blondie and Dagwood:

The game begins with a player jumping in.

> Blondie and Dagwood went to town,
> Blondie bought an evening gown.
> Dagwood bought the paper,
> And this is what it said:

> Close your eyes and count to ten,
> If you miss, take an end!
> One, two, three, four, five, six, seven, eight,
>   nine, ten!

The skipper jumps with eyes closed as the rope is turned very fast. If the skipper makes it to "ten" without missing, he or she jumps out, ready to jump for the next game. If the skipper misses, he or she must take an end of the rope for the next game.

Ice Cream Soda

Game begins with a player jumping in.

> Ice cream soda, cherry on the top,
> Who's your boyfriend [or girlfriend]—I forgot.
> A, B, C, D, E, F, G, H . . .

The rope is turned very fast. The letter the skipper stumbles on is the boyfriend's (or girlfriend's) initial.

Group Skipping Games

Peter and Paul (two skippers)

> Two little dickie birds sittin' on the wall, [two
>   skippers jump in]
> One named Peter, one named Paul. [each
>   skipper waves at a name]
> Fly away, Peter, fly away, Paul, [the skippers exit
>   when their names are called]

Don't come back till your birthday's called!
January, February, March, April . . . [players
jump back in when their birthday months are
    called]
Now fly away, fly away, fly away all! [both
    skippers jump out]

Coffee and Tea (at least three skippers; fun with a whole lineup)
The game begins with a player jumping in.

I like coffee, I like tea, I'd like [name of next
    skipper in line] to come in with me.

The skipper named jumps in, and the two jump together. The second skipper says the rhyme, naming the next player in line. When the rhyme is done, the first skipper jumps out and joins the end of the line, and the named skipper jumps in. This goes on until someone makes a mistake.

All in Together Girls, (at least two skippers; the maximum number is however many can jump at once)
The game begins with the players waiting outside the turning rope.

All in together, girls,
It's fine weather, girls.
When is your birthday?
Please jump in.

January, February, March, April . . . [players
  jump in when their birthday month is called]
All out together, girls,
It's fine weather, girls.
When is your birthday?
Please jump out.
One, two, three, four, five, six, seven . . .
[skippers jump out on their birthday day]

Tiny Tim (four skippers)

The game begins with one player jumping in.

I had a little puppy, his name was Tiny Tim
I put him in the bathtub, to see if he could
  swim.
He drank up all the water, he ate a bar of soap.
The next thing you know he had a bubble in
  his throat!
In came the doctor, [second skipper jumps in]
In came the nurse, [third skipper jumps in]
In came the lady with the alligator purse.
  [fourth skipper jumps in]
Out went the doctor, [second skipper jumps
  out]
Out went the nurse, [third skipper jumps out]
Out went the lady with the alligator purse.
  [fourth skipper jumps out]

Action songs
These songs work best as single-skipper games. The skipper must perform the actions described in the songs without missing a beat.

Jack Be Nimble
The game begins with one player jumping in.

> Jack be nimble, Jack be quick,
>
> Jack jump over the candlestick. [jump as high as possible]
>
> Mumble! [make a very small hop with feet together]
>
> Kick! [kick one leg out and back]
>
> Sizzler! [cross and uncross feet while jumping]
>
> Split! [jump so your feet go out as far from each other as possible, trying to do the splits while jumping]
>
> Pop-ups [jump as high as possible]
>
> Ten to one: hit it!
>
> Ten, nine, eight, seven, six, five, four, three, two, one! [the rope is turned very fast]

Teddy Bear, Teddy Bear
The game begins with one player jumping in.

> Teddy Bear, Teddy Bear, turn around, [turn while hopping]
>
> Teddy Bear, Teddy Bear, touch the ground.

[reach down and touch the ground]

Teddy Bear, Teddy Bear, show your shoe, [lift
 your foot and hop on one leg]

Teddy Bear, Teddy Bear, that will do!

Teddy Bear, Teddy Bear, go upstairs. [pretend
 to be climbing stairs]

Teddy Bear, Teddy Bear, say your prayers.
 [close your eyes and fold your hands]

Teddy Bear, Teddy Bear, turn out the lights.
 [mime turning out a light]

Teddy Bear, Teddy Bear, say goodnight! [jump
 out of the rope area]

Chinese Skipping

Chinese skipping is a game in which players hop over
an elastic rope (often sewing elastic or a homemade
rope of rubber bands strung together) stretched in a
rectangular loop around the ankles of two players
standing a metre or two (several feet) apart. A minimum of three players is required: two to stretch the
rope and one to jump (in a pinch, the rope may be
stretched around chair legs). As a player successfully
completes a series of jumps in and out of the rope rectangle, the rope is raised higher off the ground—to
calf level, then knee level, then thigh level.

Chinese skipping may be played with a predetermined jump sequence or as follow the leader, with sev-

eral jumpers. For follow the leader, the first jumper creates a sequence that subsequent jumpers must imitate.

In a typical jump sequence, the jumper performs the following actions while calling them out:

1. Jumps into the rectangle on both feet ("In!")
2. Jumps out to straddle the whole rectangle, feet outside the rope on both sides ("Out!")
3. Jumps to the side, straddling one rope ("Side!")
4. Jumps to the other side, straddling the other rope ("Side!")
5. Jumps both feet onto the rope, one on each side of the rectangle ("On!")
6. Jumps out to straddle the whole rectangle, feet outside the rope on both sides ("Out!")
7. Jumps bringing feet across each other, hooking the rope into an X ("X!")
8. Jumps out to straddle the whole rectangle, feet outside the rope on both sides ("Out!")
9. Jumps away, both feet clear of the rope

If the jumper's feet land where they shouldn't (on the rope instead of straddling it, for example), he or she forfeits the turn to the next jumper. A jumper doesn't move up to the next level of difficulty until the previous level is completed perfectly. The game is won by the player who completes the sequence at the greatest height.

SCHOOL GAMES

The following energizing activities for students and teachers are from the Learning to Play–Playing to Learn school program, developed by Silken's Active Kids Movement, in partnership with Right to Play (for more information, see page 294).

Scramble

The teacher writes six lists of scrambled words (possibly around a theme) on the blackboard. Each scrambled word should be at least five letters long. Students are then divided into teams of four to six students. Students take turns running to the board to compete to unscramble the words.

Simon Sayz

Students stand beside their desks; the teacher leads the game by going through a number of actions that students must repeat. When the game is over, play it again with a new Simon Sayz leader. For a more challenging game, go through the commands at a quicker pace.

Multiply Madness

Divide the class into four teams, one in each corner of the classroom. Give each student a number (e.g., 4,5,6,7); call out an action (e.g. one-foot hop) and a number that is a multiple of one of those numbers (e.g., 25). Students that are a factor of the number (e.g., 5) must move to an adjacent corner doing the action.

Soccer Shocker
Using a scrunched-up ball of scrap paper (or balls in the gym), students perform various soccer skills at their desks or around the classroom, such as dribbling, passing, or bouncing the ball off their heads.

Indoor/Outdoor Soccer
Play this game outside or in the gym. You want to have all students playing at once. In the gym use the back walls as the goals and have half the team on the floor playing and the other half as goaltenders guarding the wall; switch positions every three minutes.

Deck of Cards
This game requires a deck of playing cards. Divide students into groups representing each of the four suits. Each suit has a corresponding activity (e.g., Clubs might be jumping jacks). The teacher deals a card and the number on the card dictates the number of times students in the appropriate group must perform that action (e.g., the nine of Clubs means students in that group must perform nine jumping jacks).

Balloon Volleyball

The teacher will need three differently coloured balloons for this activity. The class keeps all balloons off the ground by continually volleying the balloons in the air. Students may not play the same colour balloon twice in a row and must have one foot on the ground at all times. Challenge the class by adding a fourth or fifth balloon.

Catch the Dragon's Tail

The class forms a line, with each student holding the shoulders of the person in front of them. The student at the front is the dragon's head; the one at the back is the dragon's tail. The dragon's head must catch the dragon's tail, with the entire line staying intact.

Basketball

Students make a ball from scrap paper. The teacher puts a wastebasket or box in the centre of the room and divides the class into four groups. The group that sinks the most baskets wins.

Getting Loose

The teacher leads the class in a variety of stretches; arm circles, wrist circles, hip rotations, ankle circles, various leg stretches. Repeat using students as leaders;

build in movement between stretches (e.g., jumping jacks then a stretch).

Rock, Paper, Scissors

This activity is best done in a larger area like the gym or outside. Divide class into two teams. Before each round, teams collectively decide whether they will be rock, paper or scissors. Both teams approach the centre of the playing area and on the count of three present their choice. The students on the losing team must run to their end line before they are touched by someone on the winning side; if touched, student joins the other team. The game continues until all students are on one team.

Freeze Frame

This game requires a portable CD player or similar device. Students stand beside their desks. The teacher pushes "play" and students can move freely to the music. But when the music stops, students must "freeze." Students caught moving come up to the front and help the teacher catch the remaining students. Repeat using different types of music and encourage students to bring in their own.

Relay

Have desks arranged in rows. The teacher selects a

movement, such as two-footed hops, and the last student in each row must perform that action to the front of the row. As the student approaches the front, all the other students push back one seat. The student now at the back then goes. The relay ends when every student is back to their original seat. Repeat using different forms of movement.

True or False?
Students form one line down the centre of the room. To the right of students, the area is "True" and to the left is "False." The teacher reads out a health-related statement. The children decide if it is true or false and jump to either side of the centre line. Students return to the centre line after the correct answer is revealed and then the next statement is read.

Anti-Virus
Seat students in a circle. Give three water balloons and a sponge to four of the students. The balloons represent a virus, and the sponge is medicine. The teachers says "Go!" and all the objects are passed around the circle in a clockwise direction. The teachers says, "Stop!" and children holding the balloons get sick, and must turn around and face the outside of the circle, but still participate. They can turn inwards again if they are left with the sponge when play is

stopped in subsequent rounds. But if a student facing the outside gets the water balloon again, they are out. If the water balloon bursts, the student holding it is asked a health question (other students can help with the answer). If the student answers correctly, they can remain in the game.

Birthday Charades

Students sit at their desks and the teacher calls out the months of the year. Students who have a birthday in that month get up to perform a physical action (one at a time) that begins with the same letter as the month (e.g., February–the student mimics flying). When other students correctly guess the action, the student can sit down. Use the seasons of the year as a variation.

RESOURCES

Silken's Active Kids Movement (SAKM)

Silken's Active Kids Movement inspires, supports and connects a Community Action Network (CAN) of Canadians who care about increasing our children's physical activity levels. We encourage each of our community champions to start a Play in the Park, and we share resources through the website and our quarterly conference calls. To learn more about Silken's Active Kids Movement visit us at www.silkensactivekids.ca.

Teachers Resources

Learning to Play—Playing to Learn

A free curriculum-based learning resource for grades 4–6: http://www.silkensactivekids.ca/lessonplan

Right to Play, in partnership with Silken's Active Kid's Movement, has developed a series of lesson plans that offer creative play activities and ideas from Silken Laumann on how to increase activity levels in your school and community.

The lesson plans are woven together with an engaging mystery story that encourages students to think about global issues. Activities feature children from around the world exploring the countries they live in, and provide a fun and interactive way for children to discuss our rights and responsibilities to the world community.

Healthy Active Community Organizations

Provincial

- British Columbia: Active Communities, www.activecommunities.bc.ca
- Alberta: Ever Active Schools, www.everactive.org
- Saskatchewan: Saskatchewan *in motion*, www.saskatchewaninmotion.ca
- Manitoba: Get Moving Manitoba, www.cbc.ca/manitoba/features/getmoving/index.html
- Ontario: Ontario Physical and Health Education Association, www.ophea.net
- Quebec: Chagnon Foundation, www.fondation chagnon.org
- Newfoundland & Labrador: www.nlpra.ca
- Nova Scotia: Recreation Nova Scotia, www.recreationns.ns.ca
- New Brunswick: Sport New Brunswick Active Community Grant Program, www.sport.nb.ca
- PEI: The Active Living Alliance of Prince Edward Island, www.edu.pe.ca/activeliving/about.htm
- Yukon: Active Yukon Communities, www.rpay.org

- Northwest Territories and Nunavut:
  Go for Green, www.goforgreen.ca/provinces&
  territories/NT/nwt.html

National

- Active Healthy Kids Canada:
  www.activehealthykids.ca
- Canadian Parks & Recreation Association:
  www.cpra.ca
- Canadian Association for Advancement of
  Women in Sport (CAAWS): www.caaws.ca
- Coalition for Active Living: www.activeliving.ca
- In Motion: www.in-motion.ca
- True Sport: www.truesportpur.ca
- Go for Green (walking school bus information):
  www.goforgreen.ca

For Canadians with Disabilities

- Active Living Alliance for Canadians with a
  Disability: www.ala.ca
- Ability Online: www.ablelink.org

Financial Assistance

- KidSport (www.kidsport.ca) assists children in
  overcoming financial barriers that prevent or limit
  their participation in organized sport. KidSport
  identifies needs in the community, raises funds

and supports program that create new opportunities for young people to participate in sport.

+ Canadian Tire's JumpStart Program (www. canadiantire.ca/jumpstart) is a community-based program that helps kids in financial need participate in organized sports and recreation. The program is run by local chapters made up of Canadian Tire employees, as well as community leaders from organizations such as YMCA Canada, Boys and Girls Clubs of Canada and parks and recreation associations.

Playground and School Resources

+ Action Schools! BC: www.actionschoolsbc.ca
+ Excelway (online catalogue of resources for guiding physical activity in children): www.excelway.ca
+ Positive Playgrounds:
  www.positiveplaygrounds.ab.ca
+ Schools Come Alive (Alberta):
  www.schoolscomealive.org
+ Safe Healthy Active People Everywhere (SHAPE): (Alberta): www.shapeab.com
+ Skipping rope songs:
  http://satsop.olympus.net/biz/skookum/
  jumpropes/order_school.html

- Skipping rope videos:
  http://satsop.olympus.net/biz/skookum/
  jumpropes/order_school.html

Parent Advocacy

- Canadian Association for Health, Physical Education, Recreation and Dance:
  www.cahperd.org

- CAHPERD Quality Daily Physical Education (QDPE) Report Card:
  http://www.cahperd.ca/eng/physicaleducation/
  qdpe_report_card.cfm

- *Eat well. Play well. Stay well.* BC Medical Association. Request a free twenty-minute presentation to your parent group from a local physician:
  http://www.bcma.org/HealthyKids/Physician_
  Presentations.htm

Recommended Reading

Coloroso, Barbara. *Kids Are Worth It: Giving Your Child the Gift of Inner Discipline.* Rev. ed. New York: Collins, 2002.

Csikszentmihaly, Mihaly. *Finding Flow: The Psychology of Engagement With Everyday Life*. New York: Basic Books, 1998.

Foster, Emily R., Karyn Hartinger, and Katherine A. Smith. *Fitness Fun: 85 Games and Activities for Children*. Champaign, IL: Human Kinetics Publishers Inc., 1992

Gladwell, Malcolm. *The Tipping Point: How Little Things Can Make a Big Difference*. New York: Back Bay Books, 2002.

Pangrazi, Robert P., Aaron Beighle and Cara L. Sidman. *Pedometer Power: 67 Lessons for K-12*. Champaign, IL: Human Kinetics Publishers Inc., 2003

Pica, Rae. *Your Active Child: How to Boost Physical, Emotional, and Cognitive Development through Age-Appropriate Activity*. Toronto: McGraw-Hill, 2003.

Thompson, Michael, with Teresa Barker: *The Pressured Child: Helping your Child Find Success in School and Life*. New York: Ballantine, 2004.

Virgilio, Stephen J. *Active Start for Healthy Kids: Activities, Exercises and Nutritional Tips*. Champaign, IL: Human Kinetics Publishers Inc., 2005.

Wise, Debra. *Great Big Book of Children's Games*. New York: McGraw-Hill, 2003.

ACKNOWLEDGEMENTS

A community of people inspired this book—their words can be found throughout the pages of *Child's Play*, and when their words have not been included, their inspiration and wisdom remain in its pages. I cannot properly acknowledge all the wonderful individuals and organizations whose work and passion helped me to realize that our kids deserve to play— these people whose actions show me every day that positive change is possible.

I want to thank the following people for agreeing to be interviewed for this book: Father Jean-Marie Mouchet, Don Roberts, Dr. Gabriela Tymowski, Victor Lachance, Colin Inglis, Steve Friesen, Barbara Curtis, Crystal Pearl-Hodgins, Dr. Andrew Pipe, Professor Mark Tremblay, Professor Andy Anderson, Shelley Landsberg, Jean-Marc Chouinard, Patrick Suessmuth, Elaine Devlin, Chris Wilson, Bryna Kopelow, Dr. Heather MacKay, Debbie Keel, Brendan Tuohey, Dr. Ryan Rhodes and Dr. Martin Collis.

There were dozens of others who contributed ideas, quotes or inspiration to these pages. Jody Lesiuk, who conducted the interviews for this book, thank you for your dedication to this project, your disarming honesty and your outstanding writing and interviewing. Thank you to the Olympic athletes who contributed to this book, to the teachers, and to the leaders in the field of recreation and sport. Special mention goes to Marion Lay, Dr. Penny Ballam, John Furlong, Russ Kisby and all those other people who work passionately to get our children healthy and physically active. Thank you to Wynn Gmitroski and Carla Dunn for the insight you provided into athlete development. Creative House has shared our vision and brought it to life through our logo and website. Mac and Julie, you are amazing partners. An enormous thank-you goes out to Lululemon Athletica and Legacies Now, whose support of Silken's Active Kids has turned our idea into a reality. Thank you for helping us support communities across this country.

To Sandra Hamilton, my business manager and friend, with whom I have embarked on this journey to create Silken's Active Kids, thank you for having faith in me and my vision, even when it made terrible business sense. Your keen and pragmatic thinking has helped make the dream of Silken's Active Kids and this book a reality. Thank you for holding down the fort during this last year of writing, so I have a business to go back to.

Ric Young, you have a brilliant mind and a beautiful heart. This combination has helped many individuals and organizations realize their dreams of making a difference. Thank you for clarifying and expanding my thinking, for exciting me to the possibility of change, and most of all for always believing in me. Your love and respect for me have helped quell my doubts and have given me courage.

Johann Koss, you are changing the world one child at a time. You are truly awesome—a visionary, a leader, a man of enormous compassion. Thank you most of all for opening yourself up to my friendship and showing me that strength and vulnerability can live together in the most successful of lives. My friends make life better and provide a foundation of love and support that gives me courage.

Thank you to my parents and all my coaches, who gave me the gift of a lifelong love for physical activity—my mom, who took us out walking every day, and my dad, who loved playing with his kids. It is what I learned in childhood that built lifelong habits that keep me healthy and well, and that help me create a positive lifestyle for my children. A special thanks to my first rowing coach, Fred Loek, who always kept it fun, and my last coach, Mike Spracklen, who helped reveal to me what was possible for my rowing career and, in turn, my life.

Tanya Trafford proved to be the precise editor I needed—organized, thoughtful and, above all, calm. You held the vision of this book clearly and encouraged me to speak from my heart. Thank you.

William and Kate, you fill me with joy and passion. Watching you, I see the world anew and am reminded that anything is possible.

INDEX